W0082024

Doctors, Patients, and Society

Power and Authority in Medical Care

Edited by

Martin S. Staum and Donald E. Larsen

What moral and legal issues are involved in the physician-patient relationship? What is bioethics? What social and environmental factors are involved in health and disease? An interdisciplinary workshop of the Calgary Institute for the Humanities in May 1980 considered these issues, as well as health care delivery, the history of public health in Canada, conflicting "health cultures," and responsibilities of professionals on the health care team. Participating in the conference were prominent scholars and professionals in social medicine, community health, nursing, law, medical research, medical education, and various academic disciplines. They included Dr. Thomas McKeown, Dr. David Roy, Professor Hazel Weidman, Professor Benjamin Freedman, Dr. Anthony Lam, and Dr. Robert Hatfield.

Martin S. Staum, Associate Professor of History at the University of Calgary, is the author of Cabanis: Enlightenment and Medical Philosophy in the French Revolution *and a contributor to scholarly periodicals and serials such as* French Historical Studies *and* Studies in History of Biology.

Donald E. Larsen is a Professor in the Department of Community Health Science at the University of Calgary medical school. He is co-editor of Family, Health and Illness *(Special Issue of the* Journal of Comparative Family Studies*) and* Health Care Research: A Symposium.

Doctors, Patients, and Society
Power and Authority in Medical Care

Doctors, Patients, and Society

Power and Authority in Medical Care

Edited by

Martin S. Staum and Donald E. Larsen

Essays by

David J. Roy
John C. Moskop
Ellen Picard
Robert E. Hatfield
Harvey Mitchell
Toby Gelfand
Hazel Weidman
Anthony K. S. Lam

Josephine Flaherty
Benjamin Freedman
Lionel E. McLeod
Janice P. Dickin McGinnis
Anne Crichton
Malcolm C. Brown
Thomas McKeown
Cathy Charles

Carol Herbert

Published by Wilfrid Laurier University Press
for The Calgary Institute for the Humanities

Canadian Cataloguing in Publication Data

Main entry under title:
Doctors, patients, and society

Papers presented at an interdisciplinary workshop
held in Calgary, May 1980.
ISBN 0-88920-111-0

1. Physician and patient – Congresses.   2. Medical
care – Congresses.   3. Physician and patient – Canada –
Congresses.   4. Medical care – Canada – Congresses.
I. Staum, Martin S., 1943-   II. Larsen, Donald E.
III. Roy, David J., 1937-   IV. Calgary Institute
for the Humanities.

R727.D62   610.69′6   C82-094139-5

Copyright © 1981
Wilfrid Laurier University Press
Waterloo, Ontario, Canada
N2L 3C5
81 82 83 84 4 3 2 1

*No part of this book may be stored in a retrieval system, translated or
reproduced in any form, by print, photoprint, microfilm, microfiche, or any
other means, without written permission from the publisher.*

CONTENTS

THE HEALTH CARE TEAM

HEALTH CARE AND PUBLIC POLICY

FOREWORD

The Calgary Institute for the Humanities was established at the University of Calgary in 1976 for the purpose of fostering advanced study and research in a broad range of subject areas. It supports work in the traditional humanities disciplines such as languages and literatures, philosophy, history, etc., as well as in the philosophical and historical aspects of the social sciences, sciences, arts and professional studies.

The Institute's programs in support of advanced study attempt to provide scholars with time to carry out their work. In addition, the Institute sponsors formal and informal gatherings among persons who share common interests, in order to promote intellectual dialogue and discussion. Recently, the Institute has moved to foster the application of humanistic knowledge to contemporary social problems.

The Doctors, Patients, and Society Workshop was one such gathering. It brought together scholars, doctors, nurses and patients to examine ethical and professional problems in the provision of health care. The Humanities Institute is pleased to publish the papers given during the workshop as a contribution to scholarly communication. This volume will be of interest to scholars and students of Medical Ethics as well as to professionals in hospitals and clinics. Members of the general public as past or future patients will also find it useful reading.

Thanks are due to the Social Sciences and Humanities Research Council of Canada, The Department of Hospitals and Medical Care, Province of Alberta, and to The Faculty of Medicine, University of Calgary, for the financial support which made the workshop possible. As always, the able assistance of The Faculty of Continuing Education enabled the workshop to run smoothly. The efforts of Professors Martin Staum and Donald Larsen in organizing the workshop and editing this volume are gratefully acknowledged. Finally, a special word of thanks to Gerry Dyer for her careful typing of the manuscript.

Harold Coward
Director
The Calgary Institute
for the Humanities

ABOUT THE AUTHORS

David J. Roy (Dr. Theol. Westfälische Wilhelms Universität 1972) is the Director of the Center for Bioethics of the Clinical Research Institute in Montreal. He is co-author of *Definition of Death-Euthanasia: A Study-Report* for the Law Reform Commission (1975) and has written numerous articles on medical ethics. His research projects include "Fetal Research and Experimentation," "The Seriously Defective Newborn Child," and "'Human' and 'Person' as Normative Concepts in Contemporary Biomedicine."

John C. Moskop (Ph.D. philosophy, Texas-Austin 1979) is Assistant Professor of Pediatrics and Humanities, East Carolina School of Medicine, Greenville, North Carolina. In 1979 he taught medical ethics at the University of Calgary. He has been co-author with H. T. Engelhardt of several significant studies of euthanasia, suicide, and the rights of patients and physicians. This year he will be co-director of a symposium on "Mental Retardation: Rights, Values, and Priorities."

Ellen Picard (LL.B. 1967, LL.M. Alberta 1980) is Professor of Law in the Faculty of Law at the University of Alberta in Edmonton. She conducted the Health Law Project in 1972 for the Law Foundation of Alberta and is author of *Legal Liability of Doctors and Hospitals in Canada*. In addition to writing various legal manuals and case comments, she has contributed to the *Legal-Medical Quarterly* and has reviewed Canadian medical law for an anthology in tort law.

Robert E. Hatfield (M.D. Alberta 1953 FRCP(C)) practices Internal Medicine in Calgary and is part-time Assistant Professor of Medicine of the University of Calgary. He is a former President of the Alberta Medical Association and is active in both professional and community groups which have discussed medical ethics.

Harvey Mitchell (Ph.D. London 1954) is Professor of History at the University of British Columbia in Vancouver. He is the author of *The Underground War against Revolutionary France* (1965) and co-author of *Workers and Protest* (1971). In addition to many articles on French social and political history, he has recently published several studies on the social history of medicine. He is preparing a book on medicine and social thought in France from 1770 to 1830.

Toby Gelfand (Ph.D. Johns Hopkins 1973) holds the appointment to the Hannah Chair for the History of Medicine in the Faculty of Medicine, University of Ottawa. He has written *Professionalizing Modern Medicine: Paris Surgeons and Medical Science and Institutions in the Eighteenth Century* (1980) and several important articles on the emergence of clinical medicine and the surgical profession in eighteenth-century France.

Hazel H. Weidman (Ph.D. Radcliffe 1959) is Professor of Social Anthropology in the Department of Psychiatry, University of Miami School of Medicine. In addition to work in public health departments and consulting activities, she has become a widely noted specialist in medical anthropology and currently directs a Transcultural Clinical Training/Research Program for resident physicians at the University of

Miami. Her long list of publications on cross-cultural interactions will soon include the *Miami Health Ecology Project*, a team research study completed in 1978.

Anthony K. S. Lam (M.D. McGill 1962 CCFP) practices Family Medicine in Calgary and is a part-time lecturer at the Faculty of Medicine of the University of Calgary. His interest in traditional Chinese medicine and acupuncture was reinforced by a recent opportunity to observe medical facilities in China.

Carol Herbert (M.D. British Columbia 1969 CCFP) is a staff physician at R.E.A.C.H. Community Health Centre (Research, Education, and Action for Community Health) in Vancouver and Clinical Assistant Professor in the Department of Family Practice, University of British Columbia. She has contributed articles to the *Canadian Family Physician* and to the *Journal of Gerontology* on various aspects of family practice. She also has a chapter on "Stress Management by Autogenic Training" in *Clinical Hypnosis in Medicine* (1980) and is currently conducting a long-term follow-up study on this subject.

M. Josephine Flaherty (Ph.D. Toronto 1968) is Principal Nursing Officer, Health and Welfare Canada. Her wide range of nursing experience includes a position as Nurse in Charge of an isolated Red Cross outpost in the North and a staff position at St. Michael's Hospital, Toronto. Among several university positions, she has most recently been Professor, Dean, and Co-ordinator of Graduate Studies of the Faculty of Nursing, University of Western Ontario. She is co-author with Leah Curtin of the forthcoming volume *Nursing Ethics: Theories and Pragmatics* (Robert J. Brady Press). Her present activities include consulting services both within and outside Canada, guest lectures in universities, and part-time involvement in nursing practice.

Benjamin Freedman (Ph.D. philosophy, CUNY 1975) is Visiting Assistant Professor of Bioethics in the Faculties of Humanities and Medicine at the University of Calgary. His articles on the rights of patients, informed consent, preventive medicine, and health resource allocation have appeared in the *Hastings Center Report*, *Health Values*, and the *Journal of Medicine and Philosophy*. Among his other publications is an anthology co-edited with Bernard Baumrin, *The Moral Responsibility of Professionals* (1981).

Lionel E. McLeod (M.D. Alberta 1951 FRCP(C), FACP) is Dean of the Faculty of Medicine at the University of Calgary. He has been Director of the Division of Endocrinology and Renal Dialysis Program at the University of Alberta Hospital and Director and Head of the Division of Medicine at Foothills Hospital (Calgary) and the University of Calgary. He has held positions on many international and national professional and educational bodies, including Vice-President for Medicine of the Royal College of Physicians and Surgeons of Canada and President of the Association of Canadian Medical Colleges.

Janice P. Dickin McGinnis (Ph.D. Alberta 1980) is Visiting Assistant Professor of History at Concordia University in Montreal. She has prepared a brief social history of the Baker Memorial Sanatorium in Calgary for the Government of Alberta and has received a Canada Council Explorations Program Grant to prepare a monograph on tuberculosis in Alberta. She has contributed to the *Dalhousie Review* and to the *Historical Papers* of the Canadian Historical Association.

Anne Crichton (Ph.D. sociology, Wales 1969) is Professor in the Department of Health Care and Epidemiology in the Faculty of Medicine, University of British Columbia. She is author of *Community Health Centres: Health Care Organizations of the Future?* (1972) and co-author of *Group Practice in the System* and *What Price Group Practice?* (1973). She also has completed a book to be published by Health Administration Press on comparative health policy-making in Canada, Britain and Australia.

Malcolm C. Brown (Ph.D. Cornell 1969) is Associate Professor of Economics at the University of Calgary. He has written *The Financing of Personal Health Services in New Zealand, Canada, and Australia* (1977), as well as numerous articles and a second book-length manuscript on the economics of health care. His other publications include several articles on intergovernmental fiscal relationships.

Thomas McKeown (Ph.D. McGill 1935, M.D. Birmingham 1949 FRCP Lond.) is Professor Emeritus at the University of Birmingham, where he was Head of the Department of Social Medicine from 1946 to 1977. He has held numerous medical and hospital advisory board appointments in Britain as well as consultantships with the World Health Organization. His wide range of publications concern congenital abnormalities, reproduction and development, morbidity and mortality, medical services, medical education, population, and screening in medical care. Among his well-known books are *A Balanced Teaching Hospital* (1965), *An Introduction to Social Medicine* (1974), *The Modern Rise of Population* (1976), and *The Role of Medicine: Dream, Mirage, or Nemesis?* (1976, 1979).

Cathy Charles (Ph.D. sociomedical sciences, Columbia 1979) is Research Analyst with the Research and Strategic Planning Branch of the Department of Hospitals and Medical Care of the Province of Alberta, Edmonton. She has written several papers on health insurance and health policy in Canada, and has written her dissertation on "Doctors and Addicts: A Case Study of Demedicalization."

EDITORS

Martin S. Staum (Ph.D. Cornell 1971) is Associate Professor of History at the University of Calgary. He is the author of *Cabanis: Enlightenment and Medical Philosophy in the French Revolution* (1980). He has contributed articles to *Studies in History of Biology* and to *French Historical Studies* and is continuing research on the early history of the social sciences in France.

Donald E. Larsen (Ph.D. sociology, Yale 1967) is Professor in the Department of Community Health Science at the University of Calgary. He is co-editor of *Family, Health, and Illness* (Special Issue of the *Journal of Comparative Family Studies*, Spring, 1973) and *Health Care Research: A Symposium* (1974). He has contributed numerous articles to scholarly and professional journals in the fields of sociology and health care.

EDITORS' NOTE

The editors wish to acknowledge the invaluable assistance of the Conference Planning Committee, all of the University of Calgary, in particular, Dr. Melville Kerr, Head of the Department of Obstetrics and Gynecology, Faculty of Medicine; Dr. Joan Ryan, Head of the Department of Anthropology; and Dr. Margaret Scott Wright, Dean, Faculty of Nursing. Important ideas were also contributed by Committee members Margaret Carlson, Faculty of Social Welfare; Usher Fleising, Department of Anthropology; and Donald Mills, Department of Sociology.

A special word of gratitude is in order for the full support of the Humanities Institute Director in 1979-1980, Dr. Egmont Lee, as well as of his successor, Dr. Harold Coward.

INTRODUCTION

MARTIN S. STAUM

Despite the high prestige of physicians and the impressive achievements of medical research and technology, both professionals and laymen
perceive a malaise in the Canadian health care system. Certainly the
symptoms vary markedly with the perspective of the observer. The issues
so hotly debated in the United States, such as basic national health insurance and the precipitous increase in malpractice litigation, are
hardly significant concerns in Canada. Yet some patients still fear
that the hard-won benefits of health insurance may be reduced unless the
question of uncompensated physicians' fees is settled. Moreover, dis-
turbing aspects of some physician-patient relationships--impersonal encounters, especially in hospitals, insufficient information or counselling on difficult health decisions--remain problematic even where cost
or competence is not.

From the viewpoint of many physicians, it appears that suspicious
civil servants and politicians require ever more obsessive bureaucratic
regulation of the practice of medicine as well as of fee schedules.
Meanwhile patients' rights advocates treat physicians as adversaries,
while physicians cannot understand why anyone would challenge their concern for the health of the patient.

In addition, other health professionals such as nurses increasingly
demand autonomy and a more collegial, rather than subordinate, relationship with physicians. Government ministers and officials who represent
the public interest meanwhile struggle to promote optimal allocation of
scarce human and material resources amid the priorities of therapeutic
and preventive care and to ensure accessibility of services.

The topical mass media surveys of the health care malaise still
discuss minor ills of the system compared to the catastrophic prognosis
foreseen by several social critics and philosophers. For Ivan Illich,
the gadfly of all professionals, the intrusion of allegedly "scientific"
medicine into the treatment of more and more personal complaints, its
intrusion into the school and workplace, is a regrettable "medicalization" of life. Aside from iatrogenic disease, the professional in this
view disables vital individual self-help and autonomy.[1] To the maverick

American psychiatrist Thomas Szasz, the sick role is often an evasion of
problems in living.[2] French social philosopher Michel Foucault views
the unholy alliance of medical professionals with ruling elites as a
technique of discipline and domination to pry into the physical and psy-
chic lives of deviants and the disadvantaged to ensure social control.
Even when therapy or public health programs prolong life, he suspects
their motives as eager exploitation of docile manpower.[3] While historians often disagree with Foucault's premises, they do often remark that
physicians acquired social prestige and authority before they achieved
therapeutic effectiveness. Thus, present controversies about medical
power have deep roots in habits of deference preceding scientific medicine. Indeed, for Illich, Szasz, and Foucault, scientific rationality
is itself unsatisfactory as a model for knowledge about man. While
other critics debate how to promote more and better medical care, these
thinkers question the basic assumptions on which medical power and
authority rest.

This concurrence of topical issues and fundamental critiques of
Western culture led the Calgary Institute for the Humanities to sponsor
an interdisciplinary workshop in May, 1980, on "Doctors, Patients, and
Society: Power and Authority in Medical Care." This volume contains
papers presented at the Workshop, which was intended to offer a diverse
group of specialists a forum to discuss at least three broad themes:
(1) the physician-patient relationship; how it has developed, how it is
now legally defined, how it ethically ought to be, and how sociocultural
barriers hinder it; (2) the status and responsibilities of nurses or
other professionals on the health care team; and (3) the general political and social framework for an effective health care system. In the
Workshop, the participants chose to investigate the nature of authority
itself, how it has emerged in modern clinical medicine, whether professional monopoly is justifiable, the relation of knowledge to power, the
right to public health services, and the responsibility of governments
in funding health care and licensing health professionals. Several
papers focused on a subcategory of these themes, while others crossed
topical divisions. Some are academic studies, while others are the reports of concerned professionals based on practical experience. The
order of presentation of papers in this volume will proceed from perceptions of the physician-patient encounter to the broader social context
of health and health care.

In the first contribution, David Roy, a leading specialist in bioethics, sharply delineates the dilemmas posed by new medical technology.
His plea for a reflective medical ethic, formulated by both laymen and
professionals, stems from the dangers of permitting technological ability to dictate moral choice. If equipment exists, should it be used? As
Roy surveys biomedical power to prolong life, to select who shall live,
to relieve suffering, to diagnose fetal defect, and to alter DNA, he
questions an unlimited mandate for medicine to intervene in the course
of nature without a consistent ethic. Knowledge in itself generates
neither an ethic nor the ability to act upon it. The implication is
that health professionals and hospitals need guidelines for defining the
dignity of the human person, and decisions should not be left on an ad
hoc basis to physicians, patients, and families directly involved. In a
commentary on Roy's paper, Robert Hatfield, a specialist in internal
medicine, agrees that physicians value guidance from moral philosophers
and further claims that they have never themselves aspired to be moral
arbiters. He nevertheless warns that rigid policy statements could destroy the flexible response a physician must have in dealing with diverse patients, especially if their health problems are not readily
diagnosed and treated.

A second bioethics specialist, John Moskop, takes explicit ethical
positions in his paper by cautiously defending existing medical authority but also strongly criticizing specific abuses. He approves of the
recent American and Canadian legal requirements for informed consent and
the ethical codes now required by research councils for clinical experimentation. Moreover, he supports a third limitation on physicians'
power--the North American trend toward national health insurance--as a
necessary guarantee that the previously unserved or underserved will be
treated. In contrast to Illich and Szasz, however, Moskop defends the
legitimacy of "sapiential" medical authority based on scientific competence, of "moral" authority based on the patient's need of a sick role
and of entrusting health wisely, and even of "charismatic" authority as
an aid in healing. He tentatively suggests some revisions to medical
curricula and licensing to prevent further abuses of authority.

The principal subject of the paper by law professor Ellen Picard is
the legal definition of the physician-patient relationship. She outlines the history of British and Canadian legal concepts culminating in
two varieties of civil actions against physicians--negligence for substandard care and battery for failure to obtain consent. She also

remarks upon legal limitations on confidentiality. Commentator Hatfield expresses his approval of the Canadian definition of informed consent, resting on a "prudent" professional standard, rather than the American doctrine of "full disclosure" of all possible risks to patients. He also notes that patients themselves sometimes abuse relationships with practitioners by needlessly consulting several physicians in a short time for the same complaint. The result may be confusion of legal obligations of any individual practitioner and financial loss to physicians when insurance administrators refuse compensation of "unnecessary" services.

Two historians then explore the origins of present hierarchical physician-patient relationships. They choose European examples because of the advanced state of social history of medicine in France, and they choose the eighteenth and nineteenth centuries as the era of the "birth of clinical medicine."

Sharing basic premises of Foucault and Illich, Harvey Mitchell argues that in the period 1770-1830 in France, physicians helped the effort of the social and political elite to dominate the low-income and low-status artisans and laborers who later formed the working class. After much criticism of the hospital, physicians decided to preserve it for the indigent or non-domiciled sick so they could practice the new observational and statistical techniques of clinical medicine. At the same time, an idealized policy of care at home meshed with the paternalistic social imperative to instill virtues of prudence and self-discipline in stable families. Thus the elite would foster the submissive worker who adopted a middle-class lifestyle and did not threaten social peace. In Mitchell's view, physicians helped mitigate the transition to a free labor market. The "medicalization" of home, workshop, and factory also included a literature on occupational safety which placed the onus on the worker, rather than on the "pathogenic nature of economic life and social institutions." Mitchell, like many of his colleagues in the social history of medicine, generally supports Foucault's mirror-image view of nineteenth-century history in which all "reforms" advocated by an elite turn into covert forms of oppression. However, his conclusion indicates his conviction that workers could not be easily manipulated.

The other European historian, Toby Gelfand, considers the social distance between physicians and patients not from the perspective of strategies of health care but from that of history of the professions.

Using the French barber-surgeon as the paradigm case of the "ordinary
practitioner" (certified, as contrasted to an illegal "charlatan"), he
shows how they benefited from their familiarity with the social milieu
of their largely peasant and artisan patients. After the French Revolution, the numerous, modest, apprentice-trained barber-surgeons gave way
to a more unified, elite medical profession, academically trained and
less uniformly distributed throughout France. There was thus a discontinuity in professional evolution from the era of the barber-surgeon to
that of the general practitioner. A wide variety of factors were responsible for this transition, from general trends of urbanization and
industrialization to increasing popular acceptance of a scientific medicine, the rise of hospital research, and a more unified medical curriculum. Even before therapeutic effectiveness, the G. P. had more typically become an authority figure, more respected if more distant socially
from his patients, and more powerful in society at large.

Social anthropologist Hazel Weidman shows that a considerable sociocultural gap between physician and patient may still exist as a therapeutic obstacle even in the egalitarian twentieth century. Patients may
be alienated by the conventional "health culture" of conventional physicians when they come from a different health culture. Outlining syndromes found in some members of ethnic minorities in Miami, she shows
how illness is defined in a particular cultural framework. When the
perceptions of immigrants conflict with those of the unicultural scientific medical establishment, the patient may feel the full humiliation
of cultural domination and also, when psychosomatic phenomena are involved, may not be cured. In despair, he may seek folk remedies or
spiritualist aid. Rather than condemning these practices as superstitious, the scientific physican, in Weidman's view, must be open-minded
enough to define the "cure" from the patient's viewpoint and even perhaps to integrate referrals to traditional healers into the health care
system.

While Weidman outlines the magnitude of the problem of conflicting
health cultures, the physicians Anthony Lam and Carol Herbert illustrate
how orthodox medical practitioners may indeed use non-Western therapies
or unconventional approaches in treating patients from another culture
or social class. Dr. Lam shows how the relief of symptoms with acupuncture treatment fits the traditional Chinese definition of "cure," which
stresses symptomatic relief. While aware of placebo effects, he believes acupuncture has an important place in modern medicine if

administered by qualified physicians. Herbert describes the operation
of a Vancouver community health center founded to respond to some of
the critiques of Illich and Szasz. The group has attempted to minimize
hierarchical approaches to patients from ethnic minority groups or of
"counter-cultural" persuasion and to enhance democratic interaction
among the staff. Provincial funding and recruitment of physicians from
the University of British Columbia Medical Faculty have ensured acceptance of the Center by orthodox medicine. Dr. Herbert's paper reinforces through concrete examples the contentions of Weidman and Lam that
power and authority in the physician-patient relationship may be effectively shared.

Both Herbert and Gelfand implicitly raise a second principal concern of the Workshop--interprofessional relations on the health care
team. Federal Nursing Officer Josephine Flaherty explicitly discusses
the current professional status of nurses, with their attendant privileges and responsibilities. She distinguishes the dependent function of
nursing practice from its interdependent and independent functions. Indeed, in frontier emergency situations, nurses sometimes must perform
procedures normally in the province of the physician. But while nurses
often follow orders of a physician or hospital administrator, they are
accountable primarily to peer review bodies, and they usually have a
wide range of discretion in carrying out a nursing regime. She therefore recommends a sound theoretical and scientific basis for all aspects
of nursing practice and a suitable ethical code founded on the autonomy
and dignity of the patient.

Bioethics philosopher Benjamin Freedman discusses the particular
moral dilemmas nurses may encounter in carrying out their dependent
functions. As in other corporate hierarchical organizations, a nurse
may be morally obligated not to follow an unethical order, or to "blow
the whistle" on a superior. Yet there is a wide range of mitigating
circumstances which may excuse the nurse from responsibility even if she
carries out an improper order. Like John Moskop, Freedman refers to
Robert Veatch's warning about the "generalization of expertise," that is,
the unjustified assumption that technical expertise implies moral expertise. When purely moral issues are involved, nurses may bear full responsibility for their actions. Under many circumstances, however,
their responsibilities will be inversely proportional to those of their
superiors. In addition to assignment of blame, Freedman discusses
"initial responsibility" of members of hierarchical organizations. He

tentatively recommends the broadening of "initial responsibility" of
nurses in an area of their special competence, empathetic communication,
particularly with chronic patients.

The Dean of Medicine at the University of Calgary, Dr. Lionel
McLeod, who firmly encouraged the planning of the Workshop, approaches
the theme of accountability from the perspective of the medical educator.
After discussing some of the most common critiques of the medical profession, he proposes how he thinks physicians can and ought to be accountable to their peers and to society at large. More efficient dif-
fusion of knowledge, less isolation from the public, more concern for
health education, more appreciation of other health professionals, and
more careful assessment of clinical procedures are among his recommendations for fellow teachers and practitioners of medicine. However, he is
not altogether sanguine about the feasibility of proposed monitoring
procedures of office, rather than hospital, practice, and would advocate
education in self-assessment as a significant factor in improving the
quality of practice.

Public attitudes toward the physician have often been affected by
the cost of medical care, and public attention has often focused on the
role of government in subsidizing health care. In an extended account
of activities of governments, professional associations, and voluntary
groups in Canadian health from 1919 to 1945, historian Janice McGinnis
analyzes attitudes to public responsibility for health. She finds the
vagueness of the British North America Act of 1867 itself conducive to
jurisdictional squabbling between federal and provincial governments
which prevented coherent policy-making and delayed national health insurance. The most important impetus to change was the Depression of the
1930s, when neither patients nor physicians could easily remain finan-
cially solvent. Though medical associations cautiously endorsed some
form of public health insurance before 1945, welfare reforms took precedence with governments after World War II. As governments began to
envisage health problems as more than just medical problems, there was a
visible trend toward ending the pre-eminent role of physicians in determining government health policy.

In comments on this paper, health care economist Malcolm Brown
stresses the interest of physicians in controlling fee schedules even if
they supported government subsidies for care for the poor. The profession has characteristically opposed both government regulation of fees

and an increase in the supply of practitioners to control fees by competitive market forces.

Sociologist Anne Crichton provides a comprehensive review of relationships between Canadian federal and provincial governments and medical professional groups. She finds current controversy over professional roles symptomatic of general political disagreements between free-
enterprise classical liberals and centrist "humanitarian" or welfare
state advocates. Using a political science model, Crichton examines the
pattern of self-regulation by the medical profession, "patronage" by
hospital boards or corporate groups, and external regulation of medicine
by the market or by government. She reiterates charges of those like
Vicente Navarro who see physicians sometimes as willing or unwilling
agents of corporations manufacturing medical instruments or pharmaceuticals.[4] She agrees with McGinnis that the Depression was a catalyst for
national health insurance and points out the remaining ambiguities in
the system. The unsettled questions include how much professional control there should be over definitions of health and illness, access to
health care, and "rationing of services." Crichton pleads for a strong,
intelligent bureaucracy, as well as community participation in health
centers, as countervailing powers to a strong medical profession.

Brown's comments lament the absence in Crichton's paper of any general theory of the behavior and goals of medical associations and governments. He fears that the real goals of financial self-interest and preservation of power may be obscured by claims made by physicians and politicians. Echoing the arguments of the historians, he also fears the
natural tendency of professionals and bureaucrats to ally with each
other.

In reaction to the McGinnis and Crichton papers, the Registrar of
the Alberta College of Physicians and Surgeons, Roy Le Riche, gave a
wide-ranging critique of the Canadian health care system, despite his
general satisfaction with the value of the services given. Le Riche defended the role of government licensing against a Milton Friedman-type
ideal of unrestricted competition, but otherwise he urged less government
interference at all levels. In his view, third-party funding and surveillance too often distort the physician-patient relationship. Private
insurance plans, with "catastrophe" coverage, might provide adequate
safeguards for the unfortunate. Indeed, he believes that the federal
government imposed national health insurance upon the provinces in the
late 1960s without a groundswell of public demand. In his view, two

other prime causes of the current malaise are, first, the public obses-
sion with health, with its waste of public funds on the "worried well,"
and, second, the permissive society, which countenances rising financial
and social costs for abortions and for the use of admittedly imperfect
tranquilizers.[5]

The final paper deals with perhaps the most basic dispute about
medical priorities--the relative effectiveness of personal therapeutic
medicine in the face of the well-known genetic and environmental determinants of health. On the basis of careful demographic analysis, Thomas
McKeown, a distinguished scholar in social medicine, concludes that the
decrease in mortality from infectious disease in the last century and a
half occurred before the provision of truly effective medical treatment.
The evidence suggests that improvements in nutrition, sanitation, hygiene, and lifestyle changes, including family planning, were the significant factors in reducing mortality. While most of the peoples of
the world still need a vigorous attack on the sources of infectious and
parasitic disease, reduction of mortality from the degenerative diseases
affecting developed societies is likely to require changes in diet, exercise, and removal of environmental hazards. McKeown's viewpoint has
already inspired some of the recommendations of the 1974 federal
(Lalonde) report on the health of Canadians.[6] In this paper, McKeown
points out the need for medicine to be concerned with public health policies, such as the re-assessment of subsidies to tobacco and dairy farmers, and to help co-ordinate an attack on environmental nuisances, even
while physicians may be expected still to devote their principal attention to curative medicine. Nineteenth-century sanitary reform occurred
before scientific understanding of the microbial pathogens. In the same
way, necessary behavioral and dietary changes ought to be encouraged now
on epidemiological grounds even before the completion of controlled
studies, if indeed such are possible, on the causes of heart disease and
cancer. Lifestyle changes need not be legislated, but will probably
progress slowly over decades. There is also a need to re-evaluate clinical services and to balance relatively low-prestige chronic care with
acute care services. When preventive programs are properly assessed,
they may be expected to accomplish more in the long run to reduce mortality than spectacular high-technology diagnostic or therapeutic instruments.

In her commentary, sociologist Cathy Charles raises a point which
McKeown discusses in his volume on The Role of Medicine--that the

effectiveness of medicine must also be judged on its treatment of morbidity, and not just on the reduction of mortality.[7] She also reminds
us of the concerns of Szasz, Illich, and others that too many condi-
tions--drug addiction, alcoholism, child abuse--are now frequently defined as illnesses. Exclusively medical intervention in these situations, with its granting of the sick role, may not be the best solution
to social problems.

    Hardly a single paper in this volume will be uncontroversial, and
the diversity of disciplinary approaches highlights the difficulties in
communication about diagnosis, much less of cure, of the malaise in
health care. If there is any hope, though, of dissipating the widespread dissatisfaction among patients, physicians, nurses, and government ministers, an interdisciplinary discussion must begin. This volume
is a small step toward that exchange of views.

NOTES

1   Ivan Illich, *Medical Nemesis: The Expropriation of Health* (London,
    1975); Ivan Illich, Irving Kenneth Zola *et al.*, *Disabling Professions*
    (London, 1977).

2   Thomas S. Szasz, *The Myth of Mental Illness: Foundations of a Theory
    of Personal Conduct* (New York, 1961); *Ideology and Insanity: Essays
    on the Psychiatric Dehumanization of Man* (New York, 1970); *The Theol-
    ogy of Medicine: The Political-Philosophical Foundations of Medical
    Ethics* (New York, 1977).

3   Michel Foucault, *The Birth of the Clinic: An Archaeology of Medical
    Perception* (1963; translated, London and New York, 1973), *Discipline
    and Punish: The Birth of the Prison* (1975; translated, New York,
    1977); Michel Foucault *et al.*, *Les machines à guérir (aux origines de
    l'hôpital moderne)* (Paris, 1976); *The History of Sexuality Vol. 1:
    An Introduction* (1976; translated, New York, 1978).

4   Vicente Navarro, *Medicine Under Capitalism* (New York, 1976).

5   Dr. Le Riche's remarks, as well as all other conference presentations,
    are available on tape at the University of Calgary Library, Music
    Division.

6   Canada: Department of National Health and Welfare, *A New Perspective
    on the Health of Canadians; A Working Document* (Ottawa, 1974).

7   *The Role of Medicine: Dream, Mirage, or Nemesis?* (Princeton, 1979).

MORAL AND LEGAL ISSUES

IN THE

PHYSICIAN-PATIENT RELATIONSHIP

BIOMEDICAL POWER EQUALS MORAL AUTHORITY?

DAVID J. ROY

I

Power in its highest form is power over men, and
the successful maker of myths has that power within his reach and grasp. Bernard Lonergan, *Insight*[1]

Power and Authority: An Opening Reflection

The making of myths is *an* effective, but not the *only* access to
power over human beings. We turn our attention to the successful makers
of technologies, particularly biotechnologies. They are coming within
reach of a very new power, a power over the molecular sources of life,
human life included. However, we need not restrict our attention to
spectacular technologies as we seek to identify the pathways to power.

Authority has always been a source of power over human beings, even
if a circle is operative here and some sort of power is essential for
the possession and exercise of authority. The important point is that
the meaning of authority itself has changed and continues to change in
Western culture. We live in a world increasingly dependent upon ever
richer volumes of information flow, upon short-term doublings of new
knowledge, upon complex networks of communications. Today, it is those
who possess information, knowledge, and communicative competence who
exert power over human beings. The information and knowledge is most
frequently not only theoretical. Real power accrues to those who know
not only *that* a given state of affairs obtains but also know *how* to
change that state of affairs. We return to technologies and skills as
sources of power, as conditions for doing, changing, creating, for
bringing about a new, or at least another sort of, world.

That is all fairly obvious, after a moment of reflection. More
subtle sources of power may escape our notice. To escape that oversight, we recall Lonergan's dictum on the maker of myths and extend
that notion. Any form of action, any attempt to change the status quo,
calls for an idea, and at more grandiose levels, for a vision. In other
cases, we finally need a strategy, a plan. Ideas, visions, plans, policies depend upon an ability to define. Those who know how to define

have access to considerable power over many things and over human beings. This is no less true of those who set about defining what could
be, and it is more true for those who can successfully define what
should be.

The problems begin when a majority of people in a society simply
assume that what can be done should be done. Others are more prudent.
They will only claim that what can be done should be tried. Of course,
technologies set up peculiar imperatives. What is tried and "works"
becomes a "must" that is often its own justification. So we arrive at
the question: does power, biomedical power, equal moral authority? Is
power our norm of what should be done, our new norm of morality?

II

Biomedical Power: To Redefine and Reshape the Human Condition?

> ...Science has in this century penetrated to the
> core of matter and life and in so doing has given
> us tools of unprecedented power. Splendid and
> cumulative discoveries in physics and chemistry
> have provided us with a definitive understanding
> of the nature of matter. From that understanding
> has come the technology to reshape the inanimate
> world to human purpose. And now the description
> of life in molecular terms provides the beginnings
> of a technology to reshape the living world to
> human purpose, to reconstruct our fellow life
> forms--and even ourselves--into projections of
> the human will. Robert L. Sinsheimer, "The Gali-
> lean Imperative".[2]

The power of biomedicine today, its ability to effect changes,
reaches far beyond earlier, more traditional notions of therapy. Some
of the developments in biomedicine, though *technically phenomenal*, appear to be *philosophically and socially prosaic*: they simply buttress
traditional values, or so it would seem. Other developments are *ethically paradoxical*: they set up difficult value conflicts. A number of
advances in the broader domain of biomedicine are *socially and ethically
dramatic*: they promise the power to alter radically traditional patterns of behavior and relationships, to modify profoundly institutions
that have been marked by stability. A further class of biomedical innovations could prove to be *philosophically and morally meta-dramatic*:
they hint at the power of taking us beyond, outside of the human drama
as we have known it for centuries.

A. Professionalization and the Masters of Dying

   People rarely die alone today, even if they may die lonely.
People usually die in hospitals and institutions, places equipped with
a massive and complex technology capable of supporting and prolonging
life, frequently only biological life, when cures and returns to health
are no longer possible. This technology involves the most varied of
instruments and ministrations. It is not a robot, working on patients
all by itself. This activity demands the presence and competence of
many professionals, the activities and skills of nurses, technicians,
specialists, and doctors. Dying today means dying with this technology
and its technologists. *One rarely dies on one's own.* Dying has almost
become a team activity, an interdisciplinary event.
   It is a work of our times that people are increasingly voicing opposition to the medical appropriation of dying as a domain to be ruled
by medical competence and authority. The key question is: can professionals be the masters of the *ars moriendi*, the art of dying, in any
case other than their own?
   It is the alienation of the dying event from the dying person and
from that person's family that demands the setting of a balance. Ariès
has described this process of alienation:

> From the end of the eighteenth century we had
> been impressed by a sentimental landslide which
> was causing the initiative to pass from the dy-
> ing man himself to his family--a family in which
> henceforth he would have complete confidence.
> Today the initiative has passed from the family,
> as much an outsider as the dying person, to the
> doctor and the hospital team. They are the
> masters of death--of the moment as well as of
> the circumstances of death...[3]

The setting of a balance is what we could call the deprofessionalization of dying. The knowledge that doctors possess about health,
illness, cure, and therapy may well give them a legitimate but limited
professional authority that does not extend over the entire event and
process of dying. Who has an authority over anyone else's dying? The
dying person is meant to be *master* of his own dying, not the professional. The deprofessionalization of dying does not mean that we can
or need die without the help of professionals. It only means that they
help us to be in command of our lives as we live our last hours.
   Dying is meant to be an act of life, an act of communication, an
act of integration. Professional skills are meant to serve the

achievement of that act. Professional authority here gives way to the
new authority that appears in a person who rises to the demands of dying with unique and personal dignity.

B. Defining Quality of Life and Selecting Who Shall Live

Medical authority may stretch beyond questions about when and how
patients will die to questions about who shall die and who shall live.
This stretching of medical authority becomes particularly obvious when
there is a question of selective nontreatment of defective newborn
children.

One pattern of reasoning underlying a specific policy of selective
nontreatment of babies suffering from spina bifida with myelomeningocele merits particular attention as we speak of the professionalization of dying. The pattern of reasoning, not the specific policy proposals, is the focus of attention here.

Dr. John Lorber is widely known for his forthright and clear positions on the treatment of myelomeningocele and associated multi-system
defects. The criteria he now uses to select babies for nontreatment
are also widely known and quite as widely debated. A number of hospitals have adopted his or similar criteria. Others have not.

What is under scrutiny here is the reasoning he employs to face
the results of vigorously applying his criteria of selection. One of
the results is that some babies die who would otherwise have reached
the levels of intelligence necessary to the levels of communication and
human life characteristic of personhood.

He points out,

> It may be feared that selection for treatment
> may lead to the early death of an infant who
> has at least a chance of normal intellectual
> development. The data presented here indi-
> cate that with modern advances in treatment
> this is possible in a minority of even the
> most severely afflicted infants. 20 per cent
> of all 110 infants with major adverse criteria
> at birth were of normal intellectual develop-
> ment at 2-4 years of age, though all have se-
> vere physical handicaps and their life expec-
> tation is short.[4]

Allowing such infants to die is worthy of debate, has been debated, and
will continue to be so. However, it is the reasoning in favor of permitting these results which calls for inquiry here.

The first statement of this reasoning follows immediately upon the above quotation: "It must be remembered that, after early childhood, the sufferings of a person with such severe physical defects and so few opportunities in life are likely to be greater in those with normal intelligence."[5]

Dr. Lorber amplifies on this reminder in his 1975 Milroy Lecture:

> Using our criteria, some children who would have
> survived with normal intelligence will be excluded
> from treatment and will die. Nevertheless, it is
> my experience, as it is that of psychologists, so-
> cial workers, teachers, and parents, that those
> young people who are severely handicapped by multi-
> system defects suffer far more if they have normal
> intelligence than if they are retarded. Only the
> intelligent realize fully what they have been
> through, what they have missed and will miss. Only
> the intelligent will worry about the frustrations
> of employment, loneliness, lack of opportunity and
> of normal family life. Only they will worry about
> their future and who will look after them when
> their parents are too old or are no longer alive.[6]

We have a position here which says that medicine is justified in determining that the working out of some destinies will be too diffi- cult for some persons. Before they have the chance and before they have to face their challenges, they may be left untreated and allowed to die. It is obvious that an absolutist position arguing for the vigorous treatment of all severe neonatal defect is not medically or morally tenable. The point meriting emphasis, however, is that those who can successfully define quality of life wield enormous power. The power to define is more than a power over words. It may easily become a power over life. That kind of power merits scrutiny and, perhaps, some form of public policy as a form of control.

C. The Relief of Suffering: An Unlimited Medical Mandate?

It is clear that nontreatment, especially the radical nontreatment advocated by Dr. John Lorber over the past few years, generally means death for the baby. However, death does not always come quickly. In fact, these babies may frequently linger for quite a while, for a period of weeks or even months in some cases. So Dr. John Freeman asks "Is there a right to die--quickly?" and addresses the question to the medi- cal profession and to the general public.

With respect to the decision for selective nontreatment the ques- tion, more specifically, is:

> If we make that decision for a given child,
> should we not then, as physicians, also have
> the opportunity to alleviate the pain and suf-
> fering by accelerating that death?...in those
> rare instances where the decision has been
> made to avoid 'heroic' measures and to allow
> 'nature to take its course,' should society
> not allow physicians to alleviate the pain and
> suffering and help nature to take its course--
> quickly?[7]

The premise for humanitarian infanticide is admittedly complex in
structure. It would, among other things, hold that: when we cannot
cure, we may kill to eliminate suffering; suffering is a problem which
can and has to be technically solved; medicine is responsible for de-
livering this technical solution to the problem of suffering with respect to those who cannot be cured; there are no limits to medicine's
mandate to intervene in a human life.

This totalitarian view of medical responsibility is a determinant
of the plea for humanitarian infanticide. This is the concept we emphasize for the moment as meriting rejection and a three-hundred-and-
sixty-degree transformation. The premise for medical practice should
be that we intervene as little as possible in any human life. Every
such intervention has to be justified, even if this justification is
usually smoothly implied in the initial contacts which establish a
given doctor-patient relationship.

Decisions for nontreatment may in a range of circumstances signify
precisely a respect for this fundamental principle, the combined principle of individual autonomy and human interdependence. What is intolerable is that further step and a further intervention, the step of
humanitarian infanticide, which claims a totality of responsibility and
an absolute imperative to intervene--the very points denied by the nontreatment decision. In a word, the pattern of reasoning which links
nontreatment decisions in medicine with a plea for humanitarian infanticide suffers from a profound and intolerable contradiction. This
contradiction centers on the limits of the responsibility and the mandate of medicine.

However, who defines these limits and on the basis of what myths
or philosophies of medicine and human life?

D. Prenatal Diagnosis: Eugenic Power?

Amniocentesis, ultrasonography with real-time scanning, alpha-
fetoprotein (AFP) screening, and, somewhat more experimentally, fetoscopy represent four increasingly powerful tools of prenatal diagnosis.
Prenatal diagnosis delivers information about the fetus. The volume of
obtainable information is rapidly expanding. More than 150 different
kinds of fetal anomalies, including those of a genetic, chromosomal,
metabolic, and structural nature can now be detected. The use of restriction enzyme and gene probe methods already permit an identification of several of the hemoglobinopathies, such as sickle-cell anemia.
This method, along with the others already mentioned, will continue to
widen the range of prenatal defects susceptible to prenatal identification.

The development of these diagnostic techniques is rapid, and the
mention of new techniques appears regularly in scientific and medical
journals. For example, a course held at the Center for Bioethics,
Clinical Research Institute of Montreal, in early May, 1980, offered
an image and discussion of the severe, usually fatal skin disorder
called epidermolysis bullosa letalis. The geneticist mentioned that a
technique to discover this disorder prenatally would probably be developed in the near future. The very next issue of *The Lancet* arrived
with an announcement of such a technique. A fetal skin biopsy specimen
is obtained, using fetoscopy, and then submitted to transmission elec-
tron microscopic analysis. This analysis reveals the separation in the
lamina lucida that identifies this disorder.[8]

Prenatal information is power, the ability to do a number of
things. Unfortunately, we do not yet have *therapeutic power* over the
majority of the disorders we can now diagnose. However, this information does make selective abortion possible. The information then delivers the power to relieve parental and familial distress, the predominant motivation for most women in choosing abortion after positive
diagnostic results.

We cannot reasonably ignore the *eugenic power* delivered by these
prenatal diagnostic methods and the information they provide. These
techniques, combined with selective abortion or fetal euthanasia, set
up the possibility of quite thoroughly eliminating defective children
from the population. Proposals have already been made to routinely
screen all pregnant women with some of these techniques, particularly
ultrasound imaging and AFP analysis.

We have already crossed the threshold of eugenics. The availability of this eugenic technology has become an imperative for its application. That technology and its concomitant power are expanding rapidly. How far are we prepared to go with our eugenic applications of this power? Will this power become our moral norm of population design?

E. Molecular Biology: A Power Over Biological Evolution?

Amongst the many kinds of contemporary biomedical developments, one class could prove to be philosophically and socially meta-dramatic, capable of taking us outside the drama or condition we have called "human" for thousands of years.

The power to design and produce new genetic combinations sets us squarely before radically new technological options that raise questions we have never before had to consider.

Recombinant DNA technology is presently young and immature. Nevertheless, the arrival of this technology has provoked a prolonged debate on whether these techniques should be employed in novel forms of experimentation. The debate has tended to emphasize the issue of biohazards. Though frequently understated, an equally momentous issue emerges with the questions about where recombinant DNA technology is likely to take us.

Cumulative refinements and progress in the development of this technology will increase our abilities to analyze genetically and map various life forms, including human life. That information combined with suitably sophisticated later generations of recombinant DNA technology will considerably potentiate our capacities to manipulate genetic components of various life forms and to engineer genetic corrections and designs. Are we heading towards a power to redesign the genetic correlates of the human constitution, personality, and behavior?

Some would doubt that so much is at stake. However, it would be naive to assume that recombinant DNA techniques represent little more than some localized pattern of molecular technology, of prime interest only to geneticists and molecular biologists. If this technology continues to develop as other technologies have--and the will to press in this direction is very strong--then it is reasonable to claim that "man will have a dramatically powerful means of changing the order of life.

I know of no more elemental capability, even including the manipulation
of nuclear forces.... It should not demean man to say that we may now
be able to manage successfully a capacity for altering life itself."[9]

This technology raises the fundamental question of power, its limits and its norms. "How far will we want to develop genetic engineering? Do we want to assume the basic responsibility for life on this
planet--to develop new living forms for our own purpose? Shall we take
into our own hands our own future evolution?"[10]

The question of the limits of this new power inevitably generates
the further question about norms, about the viewpoints and visions that
carry moral authority. These new biotechnologies "increase the powers
of men over men, thus the subjection of men to the power of other men,
not to speak of their joint subjection to the very wants and dependen-
cies created by technology itself."[11] Who shall carry the authority
and the moral mandate to undertake this radical enterprise of redesign-
ing and reshaping future human beings? In whose or in what image will
this new design be achieved? We may one day have the power to undertake such a project. Will we ipso facto have the right and the wisdom
to do so?

III

Wisdom to Match Power: The Problem of Moral Authority

> I take it that the intent of science is to ease
> human existence. If you give way to coercion,
> science can be crippled and your new machines
> may simply suggest new drudgeries. Should you
> then in time discover all there is to be dis-
> covered, your progress must become a progress
> away from the bulk of humanity. The gulf might
> even grow so wide that the sound of your cheer-
> ing at some new achievement would be echoed by
> a universal howl of horror. Bertolt Brecht, *Galileo.*[12]

We have assumed for quite a long time that the advance of knowledge and its transformation into technology is equal to progress.
With that assumption,

> we are brought to the profound disillusionment
> of modern man and to the focal point of his
> horror. He had hoped through knowledge to en-
> sure a development that was always progress and
> never decline. He has discovered that the ad-
> vance of human knowledge is ambivalent, that it
> places in man's hands stupendous power without
> necessarily adding proportionate wisdom and vir-
> tue, that the fact of advance and the evidence
> of power are not guarantees of truth....[13]

It is also true that advance in knowledge and the possession of power are not guarantees of the ability to discern right from wrong. That elemental human ability is what generates moral authority. The greatest confusion reigns in medical and biomedical science circles on the difference between right and wrong as well as on the basis for determining that difference.

Daniel Callahan has noted a widespread tendency "to justify actions with an ethical slogan or a one-sentence general principle." Callahan has observed a range of bases upon which popular ethical thinking distinguishes between right and wrong, either with respect to personal or public behavior.[14] They include:

- *The religious school*: something is right or wrong because a religious or church tradition says so.
- *The emotive school*: feelings or "gut reactions" determine what is right or wrong.
- *The conventionalist school*: what is or has been generally accepted as right is right.
- *The simple utilitarian school*: what produces the greatest good for the greatest number is right.
- *The "barefoot civil liberties" school*: one position is as good as another. At any rate, one should be free to make up one's own mind. One should not impose one's ethical views on others.
- *The majoritarian school*: courses of action enjoying majority support are right. Legality is identified with moral justifiability.

A tendency is fairly rampant in biomedical circles to turn to law, to conventional expressions of public opinion, to authoritative statements of a religious, ecclesiastical, or professional nature, and finally, to simple spontaneous reactions as the basis for distinguishing right from wrong--at least where this moral distinction has not been completely subsumed within a simple risk-benefit or preference calculus.

Hans Jonas is a rarity in the circle of those writing on the ethics of biomedical developments. He has faced the question of the foundations of ethics.

Jonas has mentioned being recalled from "theoretical detachment to public responsibility" and finding a new task for his philosophizing. Source of the call was a question latent in the "growing realization of the inherent dangers of technology as such--not of its sudden but of its slow perils, not of its short-term but of its long-term threats, not of its malevolent abuses which, with some watchfulness, one can hope to control, but of its most benevolent and legitimate uses which are the very stuff of its active possession."[15]

The latent question is really a quest for an effective ethics for a technological culture shaped by fundamental changes in the characteristics of human actions. "Modern technology has introduced actions of such novel scale, objects, and consequences that the framework of former ethics can no longer contain them."[16]

How can one best pursue this quest? An effective ethics would have to be based upon and emerge from a philosophy of organism, a philosophy of mind, and--more generally--a philosophy of nature.

> Only an ethics which is grounded in the breadth
> of being, not merely in the singularity or odd-
> ness of man, can have significance; and whether
> he has it we must learn from the interpretation
> of reality as a whole. But even without any
> such claim of transhuman significance for human
> conduct, an ethics no longer founded on divine
> authority must be founded on a principle dis-
> coverable in the nature of things, lest it fall
> victim to subjectivism or other forms of rela-
> tivity. However far therefore the ontological
> quest may have carried us outside man, into the
> general theory of being and life, it did not
> really move away from ethics, but searched for
> its possible foundation.[17]

Jonas is seeking the possible foundation of ethics. He comes close with his recognition that ethics must be founded in a principle discoverable in the nature of things. He begins to lose his way when he overlooks the fact that the principle of man's singularity in the universe is also the principle of his universality.

Even wide-ranging philosophies of mind, organism, and nature will not, as a complex set of propositions, serve as the foundation of ethics. If ethics deals with the consistency between knowing and doing, then the foundation of ethics will have to be a principle which is discoverable as a dynamic function that delivers this consistency.[18]

This is what Lonergan has understood with his position that

> the root of ethics, as the root of metaphysics,
> lies neither in sentences nor in propositions
> nor in judgments but in the dynamic structure

> of rational self-consciousness. Because that
> structure is latent and operative in everyone's
> choosing, it is universal on the side of the
> subject; because that structure can be dodged,
> it grounds a dialectical criticism of subjects.
> Again, because that structure is recurrent in
> every act of choice, it is universal on the
> side of the object; and because its universal-
> ity consists not in abstraction but in inevit-
> able recurrence, it also is concrete.[19]

A problem may be identified immediately. The dynamic structure of
rational self-consciousness, within which moral perception occurs, does
not, in fact, recur inevitably. It may be and frequently is blocked.
An unrestricted desire to know what is right, not only how to do things,
but whether they should be done, calls for an equally unrestricted capacity of matching one's doing, the exercise of power, to that knowledge. Such a capacity may be simply called willingness. Real moral
authority emerges when an unrestricted desire for moral knowledge is
matched by an equally unrestricted readiness to achieve consistency
between one's doing and one's knowing.

Real moral authority, then, depends upon a capacity for sustained
development. When that development is blocked, lower viewpoints emerge
as the only reasonable ones and bias dominates the moral scene. On
this level of perception, it is the attainment of a higher viewpoint
that is needed. But, what happens when higher viewpoints are not desired? It would indeed appear that higher viewpoints, as the norms of
morality, are a concrete possibility "only as a consequence of an actual
higher integration" of human living.[20]

The question in the title of this paper, then, leads to more profound questions. Power, of itself, does not equal or deliver moral
authority. Real moral authority emerges when an unrestricted desire to
know what is right is matched by an unrestricted willingness to act
consistently with that knowledge. Any restriction on these two capacities is a restriction of moral authority. How, then, do we arrive at
those higher integrations of human living that condition the emergence
of the higher viewpoints required to match our power? How can we possibly manage to arrive at a sustained development of rational self-
consciousness, in ourselves and within the community?

NOTES

1   Bernard Lonergan, *Insight. A Study of Human Understanding* (New York: Longman, 1958), p. 543.

2   Robert L. Sinsheimer, "The Galilean Imperative," in *Recombinant DNA*, edited by John Richards (New York: Academic Press, 1978), p. 21.

3   Philippe Ariès, *Western Attitudes Towards Death: From the Middle Ages to the Present* (Baltimore: The Johns Hopkins University Press, 1974), p. 89.

4   John Lorber, "Results of Treatment of Myelomeningocele," *Developmental Medicine and Child Neurology*, 13 (1971), 300.

5   *Ibid.*

6   John Lorber, "Ethical Problems in the Management of Myelomeningocele and Hydrocephalus," *Journal of the Royal College of Physicians*, 10, no. 1, (1975), 54.

7   John M. Freeman, M. D., "Is There a Right to Die - Quickly?" *Journal of Pediatrics*, 80, no. 5, (1972), 905.

8   C. H. Rodeck, R. A. J. Eady, and C. M. Gosden, "Prenatal Diagnosis of Epidermolysis Bullosa letalis," *The Lancet*, (1980) no. 1, pp. 949-952.

9   Prof. Shaw Livermore quoted in: William Bennett, and Joel Guerin, "Science that Frightens Scientists. The Great Debate over DNA," *The Atlantic Monthly* (Feb. 1977), p. 59.

10   Robert L. Sinsheimer, "Troubled Dawn for Genetic Engineering," *New Scientist* (16 Oct., 1975), p. 150.

11   Hans Jonas, "Biological Engineering - A Preview," Ch. 7 of *Philosophical Essays. From Ancient Creed to Technological Man* (Englewood, New Jersey: Prentice-Hall, Inc., 1974), p. 144.

12   Bertolt Brecht, *Galileo - A Play by Bertolt Brecht.* English Version by Charles Laughton: (New York: Grove Press, 1966).

13   Bernard Lonergan, *Insight*, p. 549.

14   Daniel Callahan, "Normative Ethics and Public Morality in the Life Sciences," *The Humanist* (Sept/Oct., 1972), p. 5.

15   Hans Jonas, "Introduction," *Philosophical Essays*, p. xvi.

16   Hans Jonas, "Technology and Responsibility: Reflections on The New Tasks of Ethics," Ch. 1, *Philosophical Essays*, p. 8.

17 Hans Jonas, "Epilogue. Nature and Ethics," *The Phenomenon of Life:
    Towards a Philosophical Biology*. (New York: Harper & Row, 1966;
    paperback edition, New York: Dell Publishing Co., 1968), p. 284.

18 Bernard Lonergan, *Insight*, pp. 600-602.

19 *Ibid.*, p. 604.

20 *Ibid.*, p. 633.

THE NATURE AND LIMITS OF THE PHYSICIAN'S AUTHORITY

JOHN C. MOSKOP

The past two decades have witnessed a growing number of moral, legal, and political challenges to the traditional authority of North American physicians over their professional activity. These challenges have inspired a shift in the role and authority of physicians away from the strongly paternalistic model prevalent in the first half of this century toward a more open and flexible relationship with patients. The movement toward a more equal relationship between physician and patient is occurring gradually and is still far from complete or universal; it is an evolutionary, not a revolutionary, change. For the more radical critics of the health care establishment, therefore, the recent shift in the role of the physician is not nearly far-reaching enough. These critics recommend a much stricter limitation of the physician's authority, including abandonment of medical licensing, of standards of care dictated by physicians, and of the physician's authority to certify illness.

In this paper, I would like to explore a few of the reasons for and against ascribing special authority to physicians. First, I will recall the physician's traditional claim to authority and the justifications offered for that claim. Second, I will review several recent and important causes of change in the physician's role. Finally, I will consider a proposal for a radical reduction of the physician's authority and offer some conjectures about how that proposal would affect the delivery of health care.

I

Aesculapian Authority

For centuries, physicians have claimed and attempted to secure authority over two important areas of medicine--namely, admission into the profession and the therapeutic relationship itself. These claims have often taken the following form: first, only those who possess a certain body of knowledge and certain attitudes should be recognized as physicians and allowed to practice medicine; second, physicians should have

freedom in structuring their relationships with patients so as to secure
the proper medical benefits for the patient.[1]

Social responses to these claims have varied considerably in different cultures and eras. The role of medical practitioners in *archaic*
societies, for example, was closely linked with the performance of magi-
coreligious rituals, and even these supernatural healing functions were
shared with the relatives and friends of the sick person.[2] *Western* medicine in the eighteenth and nineteenth centuries was characterized by
intense competition between different schools of physicians, each claiming to possess the one "true" theory of medicine, as well as between
physicians and other practitioners, such as surgeons and apothecaries.
Medical orthodoxies were licensed by legislatures both in England and in
North America during this era. Without evidence that orthodox treatment
was any more efficacious or safer than heterodox treatment, however,
licensure laws were repealed or fell into disuse in many jurisdictions.[3]
In Ontario, for example, no less than five different medical licensure
laws were passed between the years 1795 and 1869.[4]

It was not until the first two decades of the twentieth century
that the claims of *allopathic* physicians to authority over who should
practice medicine and how medicine should be practiced were generally
recognized and formally established in Canada and the United States. No
doubt these successes derived largely from the increased therapeutic
benefits physicians were then able to demonstrate. Also very important,
however, were political efforts organized by the American and Canadian
Medical Associations and state and provincial medical societies.[5] These
efforts led to the establishment of strict standards for medical education, the creation of state licensing boards composed exclusively of
allopathic physicians, and the protection of solo, fee-for-service
practice against alternative modes of organization.[6] These developments
gave organized medicine state-supported and virtually unassailable authority over the growth of the profession and the nature of its work.

Several reasons are traditionally cited for the authority claimed
by physicians generally, and formally granted to North American physicians early in this century. British scholar T. T. Paterson, for example, recognizes three elements within what he calls the "Aesculapian
authority" of physicians, and three corresponding sources of that authority.[7] The *sapiential* authority of physicians is based on their
knowledge and expertise within the field of medicine. Their *moral* authority is based on a professional commitment to act in the best

interests of the patient. Finally, the *charismatic* authority of the
physician, which has its roots in the prescientific unity of medicine
and religion, is based on the seriousness and mysteriousness of the
forces of disease and death against which the physician struggles. In
short, Paterson grounds the physician's authority over the therapeutic
encounter on medical knowledge, on a pledge to act for the good of the
patient, and on experience with ultimate human concerns of life and
death. Each one of these grounds of Aesculapian authority has been subjected to serious challenge in recent years. Let us turn now to some of
the reasons for that challenge and to recent changes in the physician's
authority.

II

The Patient's Rights Movement

In contrast to the support for professional *authority* exhibited in
the first part of this century, the last twenty years have seen a growing public concern for the rights of *patients* and for corresponding
professional *obligations*. Manifestations of this concern are both widespread and varied--think, for example, of patient's bills of rights, the
growing number of malpractice suits in the United States, new organizations devoted to the welfare of often neglected groups such as the retarded and the terminally ill, and legislative attempts to slow the rise
of health care costs. I will attempt to illustrate several recent
changes in the physician's role by focusing on three important developments of the sixties and seventies--namely, informed consent, the protection of human subjects of biomedical research, and government payment
for medical services.

Prior to the 1960 court decisions in the cases of *Natanson v.
Kline*[8] and *Mitchell v. Robinson*,[9] American physicians had very broad authority over the choice of treatment and the way in which patients were
informed about their treatment. These decisions were the first to
establish a clear common law duty of the physician to disclose not only
the nature of a proposed medical treatment, but also any serious risks
associated with the treatment. They also had the practical effect of
stimulating a rash of informed consent claims.[10] A similar precedent
requiring disclosure of risks was established in Canada by the 1965 case
of *Halushka v. University of Saskatchewan*.[11] These and subsequent cases
articulate in various ways physicians' duties regarding *when* information
must be disclosed, *what* information must be disclosed, and *from whom*

consent for treatment must be obtained. Two standards of disclosure are
now operating in North America. The older and more common standard is a
professional one, whereby disclosure is compared with the customary
practice of similarly situated physicians. A newer standard, first recognized in the 1972 case *Canterbury v. Spence*[12] and later adopted in a
number of other U. S. jurisdictions, requires disclosure of *all material*
risks of the proposed treatment, that is, all risks which a reasonable
person in the patient's position would consider significant in reaching
a decision to accept or refuse treatment.

The doctrine of informed consent developed out of the traditional
legal rubric of "assault and battery," based on Judge Cardozo's now
famous observation that "every human being of adult years and sound mind
has a right to determine what shall be done with his own body; and a
surgeon who performs an operation without his patient's consent commits
an assault, for which he is liable in damages...."[13] Modern decisions
have recognized that in order for patients to give a genuine consent to
medical treatment, they must be informed of the expected risks and benefits of the treatment and they must have the final decision regarding
what is to be done.

The growing recognition of the patient's right to active participation in treatment decisions has inspired a number of objections to the
traditional notion of Aesculapian authority. The *moral* authority of
physicians has been challenged on the grounds that it overlooks both
the differences between physicians and patients and the self-determination of patients. Even if physicians do seek the best for their patients, it is entirely possible that they and their patients will have
very different ideas about what is in fact best for the patients,
especially if physicians and patients exhibit significant cultural and
socioeconomic differences as well. In such cases of disagreement, respect for the patient's right of self-determination would require that
the patient's choice of what is best for him or her be honored over that
of the physician.

Proponents of the physician's *sapiential* authority have often argued that physicians should make therapeutic decisions for the patient
because they *know* better than the patient what *is* in the patient's best
interests (as opposed to what the patient desires). Robert Veatch, however, has argued that the physician's appeal to expertise in medicine
cannot justify what he calls the "generalization of expertise."[14] That
is, it is erroneous to assume that an individual with medical expertise

also has expertise in making value judgments or moral decisions. But
treatment decisions *are* largely value judgments, since they must involve
the weighing of patient values like life, health, and physical and
mental capacity and disvalues like pain, death, disability, and disfigurement. Sometimes these value judgments are obvious, as, for example, when a life-threatening disease can be cured by a safe, effective, and painless treatment. Often, however, they are extremely difficult and sensitive, as, for instance, the decision whether a possible
increase in life expectancy is worth the disfigurement of a radical mas-
tectomy or the prolonged discomforts of cancer chemotherapy. Thus, because physicians cannot claim special expertise in making value judgments, they cannot justify special control over the choice of treatment.

A second development of major importance for medicine in the last
twenty years has been the establishment of regulations for the protection of human subjects of biomedical research. Despite the grisly revelation of research conducted on human subjects by the Nazis and the publication of the Nuremberg Code, there was little or no formal oversight
of research involving human subjects in North America until the mid-
nineteen-sixties. Despite a tremendous increase in the amount of research conducted in the fifties and sixties, the issue of the proper
treatment of research subjects was not widely discussed until 1966. In
that year, Dr. Henry Beecher published an article in the *New England
Journal of Medicine* citing twenty-two allegedly unethical studies drawn
from the current literature.[15] This article aroused a storm of criticism and controversy over the ethicality of various studies. Also in
1966, the U. S. National Institutes of Health and the Medical Research
Council of Canada began to require that all research projects submitted
to those agencies be reviewed by institutional committees for ethical
acceptability.[16] Largely in response to news of another highly ques-
tionable research project, the Tuskeegee syphilis study conducted by the
U. S. Public Health Service, Congress created, in 1974, a National Commission for the Protection of Human Subjects of Biomedical and Behavioral Research to study how best to protect the interests of human subjects
of research.[17] The Secretary of Health, Education, and Welfare was em-
powered to promulgate federal regulations for the protection of human
subjects based on the recommendations of this commission. Both the
current U. S. regulations, last revised in 1978,[18] and the Ethical Considerations on Research involving Human Subjects published by the Medical Research Council of Canada in 1978,[19] require review of all research

conducted by federally supported institutions in order to determine
(among other things) whether subjects will be at risk, whether there is
an appropriate ratio of benefits to risks, and whether informed consent
will be obtained. In addition, only limited types of research may be
performed on special subject groups such as pregnant women, fetuses,
and prisoners.

Though it does not directly affect all physicians, the regulation of
medical research places new obligations on many physician-investigators
and suggests additional limits on the physician's Aesculapian authority.
Research calls into question the physician's *moral* authority in several
ways. First of all, the requirements of research design and not solely
the patient-subject's best interests must in part determine the physician's actions. Moreover, whether adequate precautions have been taken
to protect the subject's interests is determined not by the physician
him or herself, but by the institutional review board or ethics review
committee. Finally, the evidence of injuries suffered by human subjects
in risky research projects of recent years suggests that the unwavering
commitment of physicians to the good of their patients is not universal.

Committee review of research also limits the sapiential authority
of physician-investigators. Not only the concern of physicians for the
welfare of their patient-subjects, but also their estimation of the
probable benefits and risks of the research and their competency to
carry out the research successfully must be approved by the review committee.

A third cause of change in the role of the physician was the development of direct subsidization of health care services. In this area
of reform, Canada has assumed a clear position of leadership in North
America. Following the pioneer programs of the province of Saskatchewan,
the Canadian government enacted the Hospital Insurance and Diagnostic
Services Act in 1957 to provide national funds for provincial hospital
insurance programs and the Medical Care Act in 1966 to provide similar
support for comprehensive medical insurance programs.[20] Provincial
health insurance programs now cover virtually the total population of
Canada.[21] After a long and bitter battle with organized medicine, public financing of medical care for the elderly and for the poor was first
established in the United States in 1965 thorugh the Medicare and Medicaid programs.[22] Despite dozens of legislative proposals introduced during the seventies, however, the United States still remains without a
system of comprehensive national health insurance, and, given the

current budgetary mood of Congress, none is likely to be enacted in the
near future.

In contrast to the English model, federal health insurance programs
adopted in North America were not designed to change the structure of
medical practice or to interfere with the authority of physicians, but
only to pay for medical care on the traditional fee-for-service basis.
In fact, however, these programs have brought important changes to medical practice in the last two decades. In an attempt to control costs,
government agencies limit reimbursement amounts, specify which services
are covered, and encourage pre-payment group practice through special
subsidies and protections. These agencies also review the quality of
care provided by monitoring the amount and kinds of services provided by
individual physicians and investigating those physicians whose pattern
of practice is significantly deviant from the norm.[23]

The increase in governmental involvement with health care poses
still further questions for the notion of Aesculapian authority. It
suggests, for example, that the scope of the physician's *moral* authority
may be too narrow. That is, the concern of physicians for the good of
their patients may conflict with concern for the good of those needier
individuals *who have no access to medical care*. Only through social and
political action, therefore, can the benefits of medical care be made
available to previously unserved or underserved groups of citizens.
Governmental initiatives in providing health care also raise the question whether physician control over the social organization of medical
care is another kind of generalization of expertise. That is, the medical expertise of physicians does not appear to give them special insight
into how the health needs of *populations* can best be satisfied. Moreover, the physician's interest in maintaining a particular kind of practice does not appear to be any more vital than the interests of other
persons in securing access to health services.

My purpose in providing the foregoing review of recent developments
in medicine has been to illustrate several ways in which the physician's
authority has been limited and the reasons for that limitation. Of
course, interest in informed consent, the protection of human subjects
of biomedical research and the equitable allocation of health care, and
even the existence of legal requirements in these areas, does not guarantee their acceptance in everyday medical practice. In fact, these formal
"rights" of patients may not be generally respected for some time to
come.

I recognize, too, that advocacy for these concepts can be carried too far. For example, too great an emphasis on conforming to patients' wishes may cause physicians to attend less carefully to a patient's ability to provide a genuine consent.[24] Regulations designed to protect human subjects of research may interfere with worthwhile and harmless research on trivial grounds.[25] Too great a governmental involvement in health care may bring with it all of the dehumanizing effects of modern bureaucracy.[26] Despite possible dangers, however, I believe that these reforms are firmly based on fundamental human values of autonomy and dignity, and that reasoned efforts in their behalf should have our strong support.

III

Abolishing the Physician's Authority

A number of outspoken critics of North American medicine would, I am sure, contend that the reforms of the physician's role I have just outlined are much too conservative and that they already concede too much authority to the physician. These critics argue that *all* state-sanctioned support of the physician's authority should be abolished. Let us consider this perspective as articulated by two of its most well-known and most prolific adherents, Ivan Illich and Thomas Szasz.[27]

Illich and Szasz differ in important ways; for example, Illich appears committed to some form of communitarian socialism while Szasz is vehemently anti-Communistic. With regard to medicine, however, their views are remarkably similar. Both strongly emphasize the importance of individual freedom and individual responsibility for maintaining health. They argue that the individual's ability to care for himself is inhibited by organized medicine and that, as a result, medicine must be deprived of its state-approved status and functions. Both compare medicine with religion and argue that state support for medicine is as dangerous as governmental establishment of religious belief. Thus, Illich writes: "The medical *clergy* can be controlled only if the law is used to restrict and disestablish its monopoly on deciding what constitutes disease, who is sick, and what ought to be done to him or her."[28] Similarly, Szasz asserts: "it is respect for the cure of bodies (and 'minds'), embraced and practiced freely or not at all, that inspires me to urge that we deprive clinicians of *secular* power."[29]

Putting an end to state support for medicine would have many consequences. Among the present practices and institutions which would be abolished, Szasz lists the following: medical licensure, state-recognized standards of practice, state support for and control over medical education, the use of prescriptions to limit access to drugs, the physician's role in certifying illness and incompetence, and state payment for medical services.[30] In short, physicians, and all other healers, would work without state-granted status of any kind.

Given the present political power and public esteem of physicians, the changes proposed by Szasz and Illich are not likely in the foreseeable future. Nevertheless, their criticisms have focused attention on medicine's excesses, and Szasz's writings have had tremendous influence on one medical specialty, psychiatry, over the last twenty years. Let us, therefore, consider several grounds for the changes in the physician's status proposed by Szasz and Illich.

For Illich and Szasz, the most urgent reason for denying the physician's authority is the need for individuals to become more autonomous, both in preserving health and in living with illness. In placing such a high priority on individual freedom, however, Illich and Szasz appear to be flying in the face of important facts about illness and the human condition. According to sociologists, one of the most important functions of physicians is their act of conferring the sick role and thereby temporarily excusing an individual from carrying out his or her normal social responsibilities. This act recognizes that ascribing autonomy and responsibility to individuals is not always appropriate; it does not always indicate a respect for their situation and their needs. Rather, this act acknowledges that ill persons are compromised in their ability to function for themselves by conditions beyond their present control and, thus, may require assistance in returning to their former state of wholeness. Regarding seriously ill individuals, at least, the exhortations to freedom of Szasz and Illich are as inappropriate as exhorting a paraplegic to get up and walk.

The emphasis of Szasz and Illich on individual responsibility for health gives the impression that health can be secured or lost through individual efforts. Certainly, much *can* be done by individuals to maintain health, but too single-minded a focus on this fact tends to underestimate or ignore the pervasive *social* causes of illness. Because many of the causes of ill health as, for example, unsafe working conditions, poor living conditions, and lack of access to basic child care and health care, are at least partly social in nature, *social* and not just individual action is necessary to overcome them. Illich, to his credit, does recognize these social aspects of illness. His rather utopian response to them, however, is a call for a thoroughgoing de-industrialization of society in order to permit the more authentic values of a life of simple self-reliance to re-emerge.[31]

One way to interpret the rejection by Szasz and Illich of the physician's authority is to view it as a strong repudiation of the traditional sapiential, moral, and charismatic grounds for that authority. Despite the changes in the physician's role I have already discussed, I question whether, in fact, Szasz and Illich are right in supposing that the traditional grounds for the physician's authority are now bankrupt. In other words, it is not at all clear to me that we would do well to abandon the admittedly imperfect security and protection they provide. Let me illustrate some of the grounds for this concern.

Illich and Szasz apparently hold that even without licensing, standards of care, or any other official measure of expertise, individuals will have no special difficulty in locating health care which is both technically competent and appropriate to their individual needs. Two beliefs appear to underlie this view: first, the claim that most health problems can be handled by individuals for themselves, and second, the claim that the presumed expertise of scientific medicine is *not* particularly effective in restoring health, and is in fact often more harmful than beneficial. (This latter claim is stated with particular force by Illich.)[32] There is no doubt that the increased technological powers of scientific medicine bring with them increased iatrogenic potential, but Illich surely underestimates the benefits of medical care in emphasizing its risks. I believe that there are at least two important grounds for a continuing reliance on the sapiential authority of the physician. First, scientific medicine has one distinct advantage over chiropractic, homeopathy, naturopathy, astrology, Christian Science, faith healing, and all other systems of healing I know. That advantage is its strong commitment to controlled testing of its current therapeutic techniques and to the development through research of new techniques. This research activity is so intense that it is claimed that approximately half of the knowledge of the physician now entering practice will have been superseded within five years. Should some other system of healing exhibit a similar interest in examining its own techniques, and should it show similarly convincing corroboration of the efficacy of those techniques in treating illness,

I would be ready to grant it a sapiential authority equal to that of medicine. To my knowledge, however, other groups of healers are not clearly committed to such self-examination.

The above argument should not be interpreted as a naive acceptance of the status quo in medicine. I do not claim that all therapies currently used by physicians have been or can be shown to be efficacious. Nor do I claim that all physicians are committed to using only therapies which have been validated or are in the process of being investigated. Rather, these are regulative ideals which are often only very imperfectly realized in medicine. What I would claim, however, is that the activity of objective testing and validation of its techniques is much *more* pervasive in medicine than in other healing systems.

My second reason in support of the physician's sapiential authority depends on an appeal to the nature of health care services and to the circumstances in which they are provided. Because the structure and functions of the human body are extremely complex and possible disturbances are practically infinite, most people today do not possess much more than a rudimentary knowledge of bodily function and dysfunction. As a result, they are not able to evaluate the conflicting claims of different practitioners effectively. This fact might not be important if medical care were a kind of luxury about which one could decide either to take a chance or to do without. Much, if not most, of medical care, however, is not a luxury but a necessity, sought by individuals who have a more or less urgent need for assistance. In this situation, medical or health services cannot be tested before they are provided, shopping around is difficult if not dangerous, and the overriding concern of most people is not to find a bargain, but to secure at least minimally competent care. The combination of all of these circumstances, I believe, makes official recognition for some kind of standard of quality care a practice of considerable social utility.

Similar grounds may be offered for encouraging the moral authority of the physician, that is, the physician's commitment to act in his patient's best interests. The patient seeks assurances not only that his physician is technically competent to give him good care, but also that it is his physician's firm intention to give him good care. Without such assurance, the patient may feel as suspicious of the intentions of his physician as he was of the intentions of a local auto mechanic on a recent encounter. Recognizing moral authority in this sense does not, however, require that the patient surrender his own moral values or

control over his situation to the physician. Rather, it would encourage the physician's commitment to *helping* the patient receive the benefits the patient seeks from health care. Without patients' trust in
this commitment, medical care would be less effective, since patients
would be much less likely to confide in their physicians or to follow
their treatment recommendations, especially if the proposed treatment
were rigorous or difficult or expensive. Thus, it appears that granting physicians authority based on their formal commitment to patient
welfare may also be a practice which offers distinct benefits to patients as well as physicians.

Finally, I believe that there are grounds for granting authority
to the physician which, for want of a better word, might be called
charismatic. I use this term with some trepidation, since I do not
have in mind either the popular sense applied to one who inspires loyalty and enthusiasm in his followers or the literal sense applied to
the recipient of a special gift of divine grace. I think it would be
anachronistic for a scientifically trained physician today to claim
special authority based on either of those grounds. Rather, I would
call attention to the fact that like the religious minister, the physician is commonly involved in events or situations of special import for
human beings--for example, birth, nudity, trauma, anxiety, disease, and
death.[33] Because physicians work in these existentially charged situations, they are in a unique position to provide guidance and comfort to
patients and families in times of suffering and loss. We want physicians to undertake the often difficult task of caring for people in
these emotionally laden situations and to discharge this task well.
That is, we expect the good physician to exhibit strong interpersonal
skills and psychological strength as well as technical competence and a
commitment to patient welfare. Recognizing the value of these charismatic elements of the physician's role may, then, lead us to encourage
in him or her a kind of charismatic authority.

In summary, I have tried to suggest, in response to Illich and
Szasz, that traditional justifications of the physician's authority
still possess a certain force. What I have offered, however, is only
the beginning of an assessment of Illich and Szasz's proposal--to do
more would require explicit consideration of some of their more specific
claims on such topics as the overprescription of narcotics and the il-
legitimacy of psychiatry as a medical specialty.

My tentative conclusion is that sufficient grounds for some social recognition of the physician's role and authority do still exist, though not as extensive an authority as was enjoyed by physicians in the first half of this century. That is, I believe that informed consent, the protection of human subjects of research, and the access of citizens to basic medical services impose legitimate and significant limitations on the physician's authority. My argument in defense of the physician's authority is not based on any absolute rights of physicians, but rather on the beneficial effects of granting some measure of authority to physicians insofar as it encourages technical expertise, commitment to the welfare of patients, and those personal qualities which enable physicians to respond sensitively to urgent requests for help.

If my approach thus far is correct, the next and much more difficult task will be to consider what particular measures, both in the training of new physicians and in the types of social recognition of physicians which *can* be instituted, will best foster the attributes of technical competence, commitment to patient welfare, and sensitivity to the needs of suffering individuals.

I have only a few suggestions to offer in this regard. One promising step toward greater protection of the public from *incompetent* practitioners may be reform of licensure laws to establish licenses for specific kinds of practice and to require periodic renewal on proof of continuing competence. This would require physicians to demonstrate competence in their specialty and to update their knowledge continually.[34] Moral commitment and sensitivity in physicians can, I think, be best fostered by careful choice of the kinds of persons admitted into medical school and by the process of medical education itself. For example, I hope that as a humanist teaching in a medical school, I can make a limited contribution toward this goal by encouraging medical students to reflect on the moral significance of their future activities, both in relationships with individual patients and in a broader social context. If it is to have a lasting impact, however, such theoretical discussion of moral issues in medicine must be reinforced in practice by clinical teachers sensitive to the moral dimension of their relationships with both patients and students.

NOTES

1   Albert Jonsen views these as the two important issues of physicians'
    rights in the past three centuries. See *The Rights of Physicians:
    A Philosophical Essay* (Washington, D. C.: National Academy of
    Sciences, 1978), pp. 8-9.

2   Renee C. Fox, "Medical Evolution," in *Explorations in General Theory
    in Social Science*, ed. J. J. Loubser et al. (New York: Free Press,
    1976), Vol. II, pp. 780-782.

3   Jonsen, p. 9.

4   Robert B. Kerr, *History of the Medical Council of Canada* (Ottawa:
    Medical Council of Canada, 1979), pp. 11-12.

5   James G. Burrow, *Organized Medicine in the Progressive Era* (Balti-
    more: Johns Hopkins University Press, 1977).

6   Burrow, pp. 119-132.

7   T. T. Paterson, "Notes on Aesculapian Authority," unpublished manu-
    script, 1957, cited in Miriam Siegler and Humphry Osmond,
    "Aesculapian Authority," *Hastings Center Studies* 1, No. 2 (1973), 42.
    See also Humphry Osmond, "God and the Doctor," *New England Journal
    of Medicine* 302 (1980), 555-558.

8   186 Kan. 393, 350 P. 2d 1093 (1960).

9   334 S.W. 2d 11 (Mo. 1960).

10 James E. Ludlam, *Informed Consent* (Chicago: American Hospital
    Association, 1978), p. 23.

11 53 D.L.R. 2d 436 (1965).

12 464 F. 2d 772 (D.C. Cir. 1972).

13 *Schloendorff v. Society of New York Hospitals*, 211 N.J. 125, 126,
    105 N.D. 92, 93 (1914).

14 Robert Veatch, "Generalization of Expertise," *Hastings Center Stud-
    ies* 1, No. 2 (1973), 29-40.

15 Henry K. Beecher, "Ethics and Clinical Research," *New England Journal
    of Medicine* 274 (1966), 1354-1360.

16 Henry K. Beecher, *Research and the Individual* (Boston: Little, Brown
    and Co., 1970), p. 13; Medical Research Council, *Ethics in Human Ex-
    perimentation* (Ottawa: Medical Research Council, 1978), pp. 36-37.

17 Public Law 93-348 (formerly H.R. 7724). Title II. "Protection of
    Human Subjects of Biomedical and Behavioral Research," July 12, 1974.

18 45 U.S. Code of Federal Regulations, part 46, "Protection of Human Subjects," rev. Nov. 16, 1978.

19 Medical Research Council (see note 16 above).

20 Statutes of Canada,]957, C.28 Hospital Insurance and Diagnostic Services Act; Statutes of Canada, 1966-67, C.64, Medical Care Act.

21 Ruth Roemer and Milton I. Roemer, *Health Manpower Policy under National Health Insurance--The Canadian Experience* (Washington: USDHEW, 1977), p. 6.

22 Titles XVII and XIX of the Social Security Act, 42 U.S.C. 1385 et. seq. (1973).

23 Roemer and Roemer, pp. 100-101; Sanford v. Teplitzky, "Anti-Fraud and Abuse Provisions of Medicare and Medicaid," East Carolina University School of Medicine Health Law Forum, Greenville, North Carolina, April 18, 1980.

24 David L. Jackson and Stuart Youngner point out the dangers in an intensive care setting of too superficial an acquiescence to the concept of patient autonomy. See "Patient Autonomy and 'Death with Dignity,'" *New England Journal of Medicine* 301 (1979) 404-408.

25 Researchers in the social and behavioral sciences, for example, have objected vehemently to regulations recently proposed by the U.S. Department of Health, Education and Welfare to govern their research. See Carol Levine, "Social Scientists Form Committee to Protest Proposed Regulations," *IRB* 1, No. 8 (1979), 7; E. L. Pattullo, "Who Risks What in Social Research?" *IRB* 2, No. 3 (1980) 1-3, 12.

26 Alasdair MacIntyre warned of problems associated with the bureau-cratization of medicine in his address, "Medicine Aimed at the Care of Persons," Conference on Changing Values in Medicine, New York, New York, November 13, 1979.

27 Ivan Illich, *Medical Nemesis* (New York: Pantheon Books--Random House, 1976); Thomas Szasz, *The Theology of Medicine* (Baton Rouge: Louisiana State University Press, 1977).

28 Illich, p. 249. (italics added).

29 Szasz, p. xxi. (italics added).

30 Szasz, p. 146.

31 Illich, pp. 262-270.

32 Illich, pp. 22-32.

33 Renee Fox makes a similar point in comments on a paper by Samuel W. Bloom and Pamela Summey. See *The Doctor-Patient Relationship in the Changing Health Scene*, ed. Eugene B. Gallagher (Washington: USDHEW, 1976), p. 43.

34 Roemer and Roemer, p. 92.

THE DOCTOR-PATIENT RELATIONSHIP AND THE LAW

ELLEN PICARD

I

Historical Background

The relationship between a doctor and a patient has been of interest to the law for many centuries. The first lawsuit[1] to appear in law reports was an action against a surgeon in 1374 A.D. In early times the medical profession was described as a "common calling" which meant that a doctor owed a duty to his patient. Others in this category were apothecaries, barbers, carriers, lawyers, and innkeepers; it would appear that it was the special relationship between these groups who had set themselves up to serve the public and those seeking such services which set them apart from other occupations. The law had an interest in protecting the public and thus legal constraints were placed upon the exercise of the duty. For the doctor it meant that he had to use proper care, skill, and judgment.[2] This accountability was found in the law of *delict*, a predecessor to our modern law of torts or civil wrongs.

However, with the development of the law of contract there came a period when the basis for liability by a doctor to his patient was founded in contract.[3] The essential for a valid contract included: (1) an intention to create a legal relationship; (2) offer and acceptance; (3) consideration (reciprocal benefits and detriments); and (4) terms which were certain or ascertainable. It was possible to find all of these in most doctor-patient relationships. The offer was usually the patient's request for services and the acceptance came when the doctor took on the patient and commenced care. In such a context, the intention to create a legal relationship was presumed. The requirement of consideration was met by the payment made by the patient for the services received. When the patient did not or could not pay, the patient's submission to treatment was found to be adequate consideration. In most doctor-patient contracts the terms were not precisely set out but were implied. For example, it was implied that the doctor possessed and would exercise reasonable care, skill, and judgment.[4] It is worth noting that a party to a contract had to have the necessary mental

capacity and thus some mentally ill patients and young children would
not have been competent to contract with a doctor. Although there is no
evidence that the contractual basis for the legal relationship of doctor
and patient was unsatisfactory, it was eventually eclipsed by the negligence action.

The "common calling" which fostered the concept of duty was one of
the bases for the modern concept of negligence which emerged in the early nineteenth century and has become the dominant force in tort law.[5]
Consequently, the doctor-patient relationship came to be analyzed not in
terms of contract law but in terms of tort law and specifically in negligence. However in many respects the two were no different, for the
standard to which the doctor was expected to perform was the same in
each and the duty to do so commenced at the time the relationship was
struck.[6]

In addition to the contractual and tortious foundations for the
legal relationship of doctor and patient there are some fiduciary aspects to it.[7] A fiduciary relationship[8] is one in which one person
trusts or relies upon another and depends on his integrity and fidelity.
This aspect of the doctor-patient relationship probably grew from the
Oath of Hippocrates and the ethical commitments of doctors to their patients and therefore is a very basic and ancient standard that the doctor was, and is, expected to meet. Specifically, he must always act
with utmost good faith and never allow his professional responsibilities
to conflict with his personal interests.[9] If he enters into a contract
with a patient, as for the purchase of property, undue influence will be
presumed although it can, of course, be rebutted.[10] He must answer a
patient's questions honestly and not mislead him so that the patient's
consent is an informed one.[11] A very important consequence of the trust
relationship is that the information received from and about a patient
must be kept confidential.[12]

The chronicle of the legal basis for the doctor-patient relationship runs from "common calling" to contract to tort law with a concur-
rent ethical or fiduciary duty. Today when the relationship breaks down
and a patient sues a doctor he generally does so in tort. However, actions in contract or for breach of the fiduciary duty remain available.

II

Legal Characteristics of the Relationship

As far as the law is concerned, the doctor-patient relationship begins when the doctor agrees to accept the patient who has expressly or
implicitly requested his services. This means that a doctor may refuse
the potential patient even when no other doctor is available.[13] Thus,
the law does not require a doctor to accept a patient although professional ethics may demand that he do so.[14] However, it seems likely that
even the most minimal interaction between doctor and patient will create
the relationship. The rationale for this is that a patient who is led
to believe that he has a doctor will not seek other care.[15] Once a doctor has taken on the responsibility of a patient he is required to care
for that patient for as long as good medical practice dictates. This
time period will depend upon the nature of the illness, the patient,
and the availability and quality of other medical care.[16]

The relationship may be terminated by either party, but this step
is fraught with more difficulty for the doctor. A patient may dismiss
his doctor expressly or by his conduct in failing to return for treatment. Today it seems highly unlikely that getting a second opinion is
necessarily a dismissal, although in earlier times it was thought that
it might be so.[17] A doctor who fails to give a patient reasonable notice that he wishes to discontinue service could be sued for negligence
by reason of abandonment.[18]

During the tenure of the doctor-patient relationship each party has
certain duties and responsibilities. These will be examined later within the framework of the law of torts because it is there that a breakdown in the relationship would be resolved.

There are a few anomalous situations which should be noted. While
the most common doctor-patient relationship arises because of the action of the patient in seeking medical care, there are relationships
created by a request from a third party. The best example of this is
the medical examination requested for life insurance or employment and
set up by a person other than the patient with a doctor engaged and
paid by the third party. While authorities in the United States have
held that there is no doctor-patient relationship in such circumstances,[19] the English courts[20] seemed disposed to hold otherwise, although they have made no clear statement on the point. In a very recent Canadian case[21] a doctor-patient relationship was found when an

employee submitted to a specific test as part of a health check-up program required by his employer. The test was performed by a doctor under
a contract with the employer. Whether such a relationship would be
found in different circumstances remains to be seen.

How can a doctor-patient relationship be created when the patient
is unconscious? To answer this question the law, at first, resorted to
a fiction holding that the doctor became an "agent" of the patient with
the capacity to request and consent to necessary treatment. Canadian
judges have taken a more realistic approach in holding that in situations
where medical treatment is required in order to save life or preserve
health no request or consent is required from the patient.[22]

We will examine next what is expected of the doctor and patient
within their legal relationship. One point should be recognized here.
A doctor is not an insurer of his patient's health. He normally neither
warrants that his treatment will be beneficial nor does he guarantee a
cure.[23]

III

The Law of Torts and the Doctor-Patient Relationship

The two most common legal actions taken by patients against doctors
are the negligence action and the battery action. Resort to litigation
comes only when the relationship has broken down. This may occur when
the doctor is substandard in the exercise of his care, skill, and judgment or when he treats the patient without obtaining an informed consent. In the former case the doctor might be found liable for negligence or malpractice while in the latter he would be liable for the in-
tentional tort of battery.

A. The Negligence Action

A patient as plaintiff in suing a defendant doctor for negligence
must prove the following: (1) a duty owed by the defendant to the
plaintiff; (2) the breach of the standard of care required of the defendant; (3) an injury suffered by the plaintiff; (4) that the defendant's substandard conduct has been the actual and legal cause of the
plaintiff's injury.

As was mentioned, a duty has been owed by a doctor to his patient
since the "common calling" stage of the legal relationship of doctor and
patient. The lifetime of this duty, its birth, and its determination

have been discussed. The scope of the duty of care includes the following functions towards the patient: attendance, diagnosis, referral,
treatment, and instruction.[24] In carrying out his duty the doctor must
meet the standard of care of the reasonable medical man considering all
of the circumstances.[25] This standard was first formulated by the
Romans[26] and is little different today although during the early common
law it was said to be based not on any abstract principle but on the
reality that the doctor was one of those holding himself out as possessing special skills.[27]

A clear statement of what the patient is entitled to expect from a
doctor is set out in a Canadian case:[28]

> Every medical practitioner must bring to his
> task a reasonable degree of skill and know-
> ledge and must exercise a reasonable degree
> of care. He is bound to exercise that degree
> of care and skill which could reasonably be
> expected of a normal, prudent practitioner of
> the same experience and standing, and if he
> holds himself out as a specialist, a higher
> degree of skill is required of him than of
> one who does not profess to be so qualified
> by special training and ability.

Whether or not a doctor in carrying out his care of a patient falls
below this standard is a question of fact for the judge at the trial and
is usually the most important issue in any lawsuit.[29] The standard is
an objective one: that is, no account is supposed to be taken of the
individual doctor's attributes; however, it must be recognized that the
subjective element is most difficult to eliminate, especially when "the
circumstances" in which a doctor carries out the care are relevant.[30]

The doctor who has been sued for negligence by a patient is measured objectively by comparing his conduct to that of a mythical doctor
described as a reasonable medical person who possesses and exercises the
skill, knowledge, and judgment of the normal, prudent practitioner of
his special group. But certain facts about the defendant doctor are
considered under the rubric of "the circumstances." These include: the
defendant doctor's education, experience, and other qualifications; the
equipment, facilities, and other resources available to him; and the
risk of the procedure or treatment he carried out.

The details of the standard of care do not come from the law but
from the medical profession itself. At the trial medical expert witnesses, at least some of whom will be from the same group or specialty
as the defendant, are asked to give evidence about the standard of care
and their opinion of the practice of the defendant doctor in comparison

with that standard.[31] While the Canadian judiciary has a discretion to
find that the standard so described by the medical profession is too
low, this discretion is rarely exercised. It does so only when the
fact situation is one in which the ordinary person could see that precautions which could have been taken were not, as where a surgeon did
not either tape or count sponges after an adenoid operation, and a child
asphyxiated. In that case, although the medical evidence was that the
doctor had met the standard of care, the judge found the standard to be
too low and the doctor to be liable.[32]

This process whereby the setting of the standard of care and the
evaluation of the defendant's actions are done by a judge using the
evidence of medical witnesses may be seen as the medical profession assessing itself. But it must be remembered that the judge has no other
way of establishing a framework within which to decide whether a doctor
has been negligent. Similarly, reference to fellow members of a profession is made when the defendant is an accountant or a lawyer.[33]
Within the adversary system there are checks on the possible abuse of
the role played by the medical profession in a negligence action against
a doctor: witnesses are subjected to cross-examination, the judge has
the power to accept or reject evidence and the discretion to find the
standard of care too low.

The patient has the onus of proving his injury and that it occurred
as a result of the doctor's negligence. This can be an onerous burden
because of the difficulty of showing cause and effect when dealing with
the human body.[34] And, once again, the patient must call upon the medical profession for proof of an essential element of his case. There
is a legal principle which applies to negligence law in general which
states that a plaintiff may only recover for an injury that was foreseeable to a person in the position of the defendant.[35] Thus, the complexities of the human body combined with the mysteries of modern medicine may mean that a patient is injured by substandard practice but in
a way which was not foreseeable. In that case the patient will not recover any compensation.[36]

There are a number of defences available to a doctor who is sued
for negligence, including: that he followed the approved practice,[37]
i.e., met the standard of care; that he simply made an error of judgment;[38] that the time period within which he could be sued has ex-
pired;[39] or that the patient was guilty of contributory negligence.
Although it is not possible within the ambit of this paper to review

all of these defences in depth, I have done so elsewhere.[40] But the
last defence, that of contributory negligence, is of particular interest at this time for it was only quite recently in Canada that a patient's claim against a doctor was reduced by two-thirds because of her
failure to take reasonable care of herself.[41] After her doctor's prescription for a drug to treat her skin disorder ran out, she continued
taking it, but her source was a drug company salesman. Eventually she
went blind as a consequence of using the drug. The doctor was found to
be one-third to blame for his failure to carefully read an ophthalmolo-
gist's report which would have alerted him to the risk for the patient.
This decision marks a recognition of the patient as a real factor in
medical treatment. Just as the standard of care which a doctor must
meet is constantly rising with advances in medicine, so will the standard which each patient is supposed to meet in taking care of himself.
This greater accountability of the patient is based on greater public
awareness, access to information, and availability of medical care.
One caveat on such an elevated standard for the patient must be that
not all patients have these resources. In any case, it appears that
the law is going to require patients to take a greater responsibility
for their own health care.

In summary, the negligence or malpractice action is the appropriate one for a patient who has been injured by the substandard treatment
of a doctor. It is the same type of action that a client could take
against a lawyer, or one motorist against another. The main function
of the action is to compensate a victim although it may also elevate
standards, punish and deter the defendant, and provide a catharsis for
the plaintiff. It may not be the best means of resolving a breakdown
in a relationship, and in the United States and New Zealand alternatives to civil litigation are being tried. We in Canada must watch
these developments carefully.[42]

B. The Battery Action--With Reference to Informed Consent

Where a patient alleges that he has not consented to the medical
treatment given, he can sue the doctor in battery. Battery is a very
old action protecting the right of an individual to be free of unauthor-
ized touching of any kind, even that which is beneficial to him.[43]

It is perhaps necessary to note here that the negligence action
has also been brought when a risk, which has not been explained to a
patient, materializes and injures him.[44] At present, the Supreme Court

of Canada has reserved judgment on two cases[45] which raise the complex
issues with respect to the appropriate cause of action: battery or
negligence. It is to be hoped that these decisions will make the jurisprudence more clear.

But the present uncertainties in the law do not preclude a discussion of the defence of informed consent. Informed consent is a true defence which means that the onus of establishing it is on the defendant
doctor.[46] The patient has to prove that he received treatment, i.e.,
that he was touched, and for practical reasons will usually go on to
state that he did not consent. However, this does not derogate from
the responsibility to prove the defence which rests on the defendant.

In order to be valid the consent given by a patient for medical
treatment must be: (1) voluntary; (2) referable to the treatment given
and the person or persons administering it; (3) given by someone who
has capacity; (4) informed.

I propose to deal here only with the last requirement because it
highlights the importance of the doctor-patient relationship.[47] A preliminary point to note is that Canadian law in the area of informed
consent is different from that of the United States. Thus, American
jurisprudence and literature may be misleading to Canadians.

Obviously, before a patient can make a decision about whether or
not to consent to medical treatment, he must have certain information,
and similarly before a doctor can make certain decisions about the best
care for the patient, he requires all relevant information. This process should be a bilateral one wherein each party to the relationship
not only has a right to, but also a concomitant duty to, provide material facts. Viewing this as a unilateral situation results in a one-
sided relationship wherein the doctor is expected to elicit what he
needs to know from the patient and is not expected to provide much information to the patient. It is only the bilateral model which is consistent with the modern legal requirements of the doctor-patient relationship. In Canada the law requires a doctor to disclose those risks
which his colleagues would normally disclose to *the* particular patient
he is caring for. This is an objective "professional disclosure" standard for the doctor but a subjective standard with respect to the patient, whose unique strengths or weaknesses may increase or decrease
the information which the doctor is required to convey.[48] Clearly the
doctor must fully answer any questions asked by a patient.[49] An entirely different and higher standard applies if the procedure is

experimental, for then the doctor must disclose all of the risks involved. This is called the "full disclosure" standard.[50]

The professional disclosure standard combined with the subjective
patient standard balances the interests of both doctor and patient.
For while a good deal of discretion with regard to what risks should be
revealed remains with the doctor, he has the onus of proving that he
met the standard. Meanwhile, the patient who has a duty to assist in
his own assessment[51] can expect to have his questions honestly answered
and the risks explained to him in a way which *he* can understand. Thus,
the good health of the doctor-patient relationship depends heavily on a
bilateral exchange in which there is communication, between a doctor
who acts in good faith and places the patient's welfare first and a patient who takes a responsible role and realizes that medical science
and judgment are not infallible.

C. Confidentiality

Just as communication is essential to a doctor-patient relationship so too is confidentiality essential to good communication. The
duty of the doctor in this regard remains today as it was in the *Oath
of Hippocrates*:

> Whatsoever I see or hear in the course of my prac-
> tice, or outside my practice in social intercourse,
> that ought never to be published abroad, I will not
> divulge, but consider such things to be held secret.

Modern adaptations of this tenet have reflected the fact that doctor-
patient communications are not privileged in a court of law by the
insertion of such clauses as "except where the law requires him to do
so." The rule that a doctor can be required to testify in a court of
law about confidences revealed to him by a patient within the doctor-
patient relationship was first enunciated in 1776[52] but remains in the
law today. Some inroads have been made into it by judges who have been
reluctant to compel a doctor to testify[53] and much research and discussion has taken place about changing the law by statute to allow a discretionary power to a judge to excuse a doctor from testifying.[54] It
seems likely that there will be some legal reform in this area which
would reflect a recognition by the law of the importance of confidentiality of communications within the doctor-patient relationship.

Testimony in court aside, there is no doubt that a patient has a
cause of action against a doctor who reveals confidental information[55]

other than when expressly permitted by the patient or required by statute[56] or when the public interest to be protected by doing so is very
great.[57]

Recent concerns over medical audits, peer reviews of doctors, and
the right of nurses to point out deficiencies in health care have seen
this right to confidentiality incorrectly described as being the doctor's. The law does afford protection to the doctor through the action
for defamation, but it would obviously be against the public interest
to cloak in secrecy the doctor's exercise of professional care, skill,
and judgment. Indeed, hearkening back to earlier stages in the law
(and this paper), the doctor's legal responsibilities flow from his
provision of professional services and his exercise of care, skill,
and judgment.

To date, there have been few lawsuits based on the breach of confidentiality in the doctor-patient relationship, which may mean that
patients are satisfied with the way in which confidential information
is being dealt with, or that they are unaware of or reluctant to pursue
the protection given to them by law.

IV

Conclusion

Because the doctor-patient relationship is such a critical one to
society, the law takes a great interest in its vitality. The minimum
standard that the medical profession and the patient must meet are ascertainable from decided cases. Although these standards are objective, they are not rigid, but attempt to evolve with medical science
and the requirements of society. While the doctor is held accountable
for the knowledge and skills he claims to possess, the law does not expect perfection from him. Furthermore, the medical profession plays a
major role in the determination of the standards which the law will
propound. For the patient who alleges he has suffered an injury or has
had a basic right violated by a doctor, the law sets up a process whereby he can claim compensation. But in the conduct of civil litigation,
the patient must prove his case against the doctor and furthermore the
patient's conduct will be relevant to the determination of the case.

Law is the mentor of the doctor-patient relationship.

NOTES

1 *Morton's Case* (1374) 48 Edw. III f.6, pl. 11.

2 Holdsworth, *History of English Law* vol. 3, p. 385; *Everard* v. *Hopkins* (1615) 80 E.R. 1165 (K.B.).

3 Holdsworth, p. 448; Cheshire and Fifoot, *Law of Contract* (8th ed. 1972).

4 *Slater* v. *Baker* (1767) 2 Wils. K.B. 359, 95 E.R. 860.

5 Fleming, *The Law of Torts* (4th ed. 1971), p. 102.

6 Nathan, *Medical Negligence* (1956), p. 7.

7 *Kenny* v. *Lockwood* [1932] 1 D.L.R. 507 (Ont. C.A.); *Halushka* v. *University of Saskatchewan* [1965] 53 D.L.R. (2d) 436 (Sask. C.A.); Hopper, *"The Medical Man's Fiduciary Duty "* *Law Teacher* 7 (1973), 73.

8 *Black's Law Dictionary* (5th ed. 1979), p. 564. Note that the lawyer is in a fiduciary relationship with his client.

9 Wasmuth, *Law for the Physician*, Lea and Febiger, Philadelphia, 1966.

10 Côté, *An Introduction to the Law of Contract* (1974), p. 105.

11 *Kenny* v. *Lockwood supra* n. 7; *Reibl* v. *Hughes* (1978) 6 C.C.L.T. 227 (Ont. C.A.); Dickens, "Contractual Aspects of Human Medical Experimentation," *University of Toronto Law Journal* 25 (1975), 406 at 426.

12 Speller, *Law of Doctor and Patient* (1973), p. 127.

13 *Hurley* v. *Eddingfield* (1901) 59 N.E. 1058 (Ind. S.C.); Godfrey, "Emergency Care: Physicians should be placed under an affirmative duty to render essential medical aid in emergency circumstances," *University of California at Davis Law Review* 7 (1974), 246 at 249.

14 Nathan, *Medical Negligence*.

15 See *Barnett* v. *Chelsea and Kensington Hospital* [1969] 1 Q.B. 428.

16 *Baltzan* v. *Fidelity Ins. Co.* [1932] 3 W.W.R. 140, [1933] 3 W.W.R. 203 (Sask. C.A.); Stetler and Mortz, *Doctor and Patient and the Law* (St. Louis: C. V. Mosby, 1962), p. 123.

17 *Town* v. *Archer* (1902) 4 O.L.R. 383 at 386.

18 Waltz and Inbau, *Medical Jurisprudence* (New York: MacMillan, 1971), p. 147.

19 *Wilcox* v. *Salt Lake City Corporation* (1971) 26 Utah 78 (S.C.); Louisell and Williams, *Medical Malpractice* (New York: Matthew Bender, 1969).

20 Nathan, *Medical Negligence*.

21 *Leonard* v. *Knott* [1980] 1 W.W.R. 673 (B.C.C.A.).

22 *Matheson* v. *Smiley* [1932] 2 D.L.R. 787 (Man. C.A.); *Marshall* v.
    Curry [1933] 3 D.L.R. 260 (N.S.S.C.).

23 *Johnston* v. *Wellesley Hospital* (1970) 17 D.L.R. (3d) 139 (Ont.);
    Haines, "Courts and Doctors," *Canadian Bar Review* 30 (1952), 483.

24 For a fuller discussion of each duty *see* Picard, *Legal Liability of
    .Doctors and Hospitals in Canada* (1978).

25 *McCormick* v. *Marcotte* [1972] S.C.R. 18 at 21.

26 *Lex Aquilia* 287 Digest 9.2.1.

27 Fleming, *The Law of Torts*.

28 *Crits* v. *Sylvester* [1956] 1 D.L.R. (2d) 502 at 508; *affirmed* [1956]
    S.C.R. 991.

29 Linden, *Canadian Tort Law* (1977), p. 82.

30 Nathan, *Medical Negligence*, pp. 22-23.

31 Picard, *Legal Liability*, pp. 195-218.

32 *Chasney* v. *Anderson* [1950] 4 D.L.R. 223 (S.C.C.).

33 See Linden, *Canadian Tort Law* (1977), p. 108.

34 See *Girard* v. *Royal Columbian Hospital* [1976] 66 D.L.R. (3d) 676 at
    691 (B.C.S.C.).

35 Linden, pp. 305-355.

36 *University Hospital Board* v. *Lepine* [1966] S.C.R. 561.

37 See *Challand* v. *Bell* [1959] 18 D.L.R. (2d) 150 (Alta. S.C.).

38 See *Wilson* v. *Swanson* [1956] 5 D.L.R. (2d) 113 (S.C.C.).

39 See *Mumford* v. *Children's Hospital* [1977] 1 W.W.R. 666 (Man. C.A.).

40 Picard, *Legal Liability*, pp. 169-195.

41 *Crossman* v. *Stewart* (1977) 5 C.C.L.T. 45 (B.C.S.C.); See also *Hôpital
    Notre-Dame de l'Espérance* v. *Laurent* [1978] 1 S.C.R. 605.

42 See Sharpe and Sawyer, *Doctors and the Law* (1978).

43 Fleming, *The Law of Torts*, p. 25.

44 See Picard, "The Tempest of Informed Consent" in *Studies in Canadian
    Tort Law* (2d ed. Klar 1977), p. 129.

45 *Lepp* v. *Hopp* (1979) 8 C.C.L.T. 260 (Alta. S.C.); *Reibl* v. *Hughes* (1978) 6 C.C.L.T. 227 (Ont. C.A.).

46 *Schweizer* v. *Central Hospital* (1974) 6 O.R. (2d) 606 (H.C.); Linden, *Medical Negligence*, p. 55.

47 For a more complete discussion see Picard, *Legal Liability*, pp. 63-91.

48 See Picard, "The Tempest of Informed Consent."

49 *Smith* v. *Auckland Hospital Board* [1965] N.Z. L. R. 191 (C.A.); *Male* v. *Hopmans* (1966) 54 D.L.R. (2d) 592 (Ont. H.C.).

50 *Halushka* v. *University of Saskatchewan* (1965) 53 D.L.R. (2d) 436 (Sask. C.A.).

51 Kouri, "The Patient's Duty to Co-operate," *Revue de Droit de l'Université Sherbrooke* 3 (1972), 44.

52 *Kingston's (Duchess) Case* (1776) 20 State Tr. 619.

53 *A.G.* v. *Mulholland* [1963] 2 Q.B. 477 (C.A.).

54 Law Reform Commission of Canada, *Report on Evidence* (1977), p. 80.

55 *A.B.* v. *C.D.* (1851) 14 Dunlop's S.C. 177 (Scot. C.S.); *Furniss* v. *Fitchett* [1958] N.Z.L.R. 396 (N.Z.S.C.).

56 As in most jurisdictions for communicable disease, vital statistics, health care record keeping, etc.

57 See Picard, *Legal Liability*, pp. 38-41.

COMMENTS ON THE PAPERS OF
ROY, MOSKOP, AND PICARD

ROBERT E. HATFIELD

These three papers provide challenge, comfort, and information to
the practicing doctor. I thank the speakers for their contributions,
which I shall relate to the daily work of the bedside clinician. All
too often the physician exerts the power and moral authority described
by Dr. Roy, without being aware of the physician's authority as carefully developed by Professor Moskop. Furthermore, the physician is only
intermittently and vaguely aware of the medical-legal threat implicit in
any written or unwritten professional contract including that of the
doctor and the patient, as succinctly and clearly outlined by Professor
Picard.

The thesis developed by Dr. Roy is intriguing. I support his contention that the communicators of today wield tremendous power, perhaps
even more than that gained by those people who gather more and more information. To wit, when the Virginia Slims mechanical model, beautiful
as she may be, vibrantly proclaims, "You've come a long way, Baby" one
trusts that she does not fully comprehend the gravity of her pronounce-
ment. Current projections suggest that from an incidence of virtually
zero, cancer of the lung in North American females will be more common
in the mid-1980s than will be cancer of the breast. There is little
doubt that the most important and significant factor in this epidemiological change has been advertising itself. The implications of the
commonly-cited figure that medical information is doubling at a
five-year rate are mind-boggling. Translated into my own medical career, the amount of medical knowledge doubled between the time I began
medical studies and the completion of my internship. Before I conclude
my career, medical knowledge will have increased by a factor of 128.
This seems preposterous, for no human being could be expected to master
such a burgeoning amount of data. On the other hand, I see a different
trend when I reflect on one tiny aspect of one medical subject, i.e.,
the drugs currently being used for high blood pressure management. Today, as opposed to when I first studied the subject, only one family of
diuretics is still in vogue along with the acknowledgment that salt restriction is an important factor in treatment.

The importance of communication as a tool of power is emphasized in several studies, not widely circulated, relating to the doctor-patient relationship. About three-quarters of the complaints regarding doctors, especially those which proceed to become formal medico-legal cases, relate to patients' unhappiness with the way the doctor dealt with them as a person rather than to a direct attack upon the doctor's skill, knowledge, or judgment.

I am indebted to Professor Picard for her concise outline of the development of the doctor-patient relationship and further to Professor Moskop for expanding upon the legally defined relationship by pointing out the responsibilities and obligations incumbent upon both parties, i.e., the doctor and the patient. There is little doubt that the practicing physician of Alberta (and probably those in all other Canadian provinces) feels increasingly that the doctor's obligations have been greatly increased with the introduction of universal prepaid medical care insurance. Conversely the whole concept of patient responsibility seems steadily to have diminished. Often the doctor feels that somehow he or she has become an apologist for government by having to explain to the patient the provisions of "medicare." It is often a shock to the patient to be told that coverage is not truly universal and that arbitrary decisions by health care commissions often deprive the doctor of income by merely changing the definition of a service. In turn, the doctor frequently finds himself defending, to the government, the need for a service to a patient or indications for a particular test. This kind of public relations work rarely pleases the parties concerned, is never paid for, and is time-consuming. Most galling is the recognition that the initial contract is between the government and the patient, not between government and the doctor! In short, although the communications professions often imply, if not openly accuse, doctors of benefiting excessively from "medicare," rarely is there public demonstration of, or outcry about, abuse of the system by the consumer. So it seems to the physician. Almost any doctor can give innumerable illustrations of this contention. I think of a seventeen-year-old patient who calmly announced to me when I was first asked to see him that I was "doctor number 33 on the case." I strongly believe that a goodly number of those doctor contacts were not necessary, and were patient-inspired, rather than thoughtful consultations requested by the family doctor.

I suspect that many doctors are only vaguely aware of some of the legal aspects of their relationship with patients, as outlined by Professor Picard. It is comforting to know that in fact the doctor can refuse to treat a potential patient even when no other doctor is available. I hadn't pondered deeply the matter of defining the end of a patient-doctor relationship, yet I am aware that this also is an area which breeds medico-legal litigation, i.e., when doctors hand over care of a patient to holiday relief doctors, night call and weekend-covering colleagues. Who is in fact responsible for a patient's care when he or she is in the midst of an out-of-hospital investigation involving consultation by two other consulting physicians, prior to receipt of the reports of those physicians by the original doctor? And what if the visits to those two consultants were initiated by the patient, unbeknownst to the family doctor, and that the consulting doctors believed them to have in fact been referred visits? These are very practical concerns.

I doubt that many doctors are aware of the fact that the principle is recognized in Canadian law that the patient must take reasonable care of himself or herself while under the doctor's care. In this era of doctor-shopping, polypharmacy, and the extension of longevity, it seems only right that as a patient is increasingly protected by a rising awareness of "patient's rights," that the doctor equally deserves protection from litigious patients. I appreciate Professor Picard's prophecy that Canadian law is going to require patients to take an even greater responsibility for their health care.

The matter of informed consent to me is at the same instant a matter of necessity and unattainable nonsense. No one can argue against the idea that each of us has a right to know what is happening to us, especially when someone else is exerting a control over our very lives. The standard of education has risen dramatically in North America in recent decades. The social context of a hundred years ago is now irrelevant. Then only a few of the citizens of any village had any degree of education at all, and others rarely questioned the words of the local "educated" people. Today, quite often the patient has had as many years of formal education and training as has the doctor, albeit in a different field of study.

On the other hand, to make an assumption that by taking ten, twenty, or thirty minutes the doctor can successfully impart to the patient comprehensive knowledge about a given procedure, a disease process, or

the hazards and potential benefits of a given drug is frequently unjustified. It would take me two to five minutes to read to someone
else the contraindications and reported untoward or adverse effects of
one simple drug such as diazepam, one of the most commonly prescribed
medicines in North America today. Even after reading the lists, were I
to satisfy what is theoretically intended as "informed consent," I would
have to further explain most of the terms, changing them into non-medical language. Finally I would have to deal with the emotional response
that each individual patient may have to many of the words. My own
mother died of Hodgkins' Disease. Were I to listen to a recitation from
my own physician regarding potential adverse effects of a drug, and hear
something relating to bone marrow changes or swellings of lymph nodes,
it would be natural for me to have more than average concern. I might
reflect that my mother died of a disease process that just might be related to the problems I was being told could result from taking this
particular medicine. Moreover, the drug might not give me the desired
effect for my condition, anyway. I think that my own medical knowledge
and years of experience would help me personally to resolve such emotional responses very quickly. It might not be so easy for someone
else. One can quickly begin to imagine the magnitude of the problem of
truly "informing" a patient about a procedure or a drug. This is com-
pounded by the fact that most people who are taking medicines for a
particular reason are usually taking more than one at a given time. Informing patients must be viewed in terms of time which, per se, is
usually poorly compensated in our medical payment systems. Finally
many patients do not appreciate contacts with doctors that seem to drag
on unnecessarily. Increasingly one hears the militant cry, "my time is
just as valuable as the doctor's."

One can perhaps appreciate then some of the agony of the practicing
doctor. I firmly believe that the great majority of Canadian physicians
want to share the knowledge of diagnosis, prognosis, and treatment with
the patient as much as possible. The practical concerns which I have
outlined make this exceedingly difficult. It is rather frightening to
sense that lawsuits can result, nay, indeed do result, when it is
judged that the patient has not been properly informed. Once again, I
am particularly pleased to learn from Professor Picard that Canadian
law has established the "professional disclosure" stand for the doctor
as opposed to the "full disclosure" standard, which I believe is almost
impossible to achieve. The whole issue of "informed consent" is related

to the wider issue of the relative amounts of power exercised by both
patient and doctor in the patient-doctor relationship (contract). Indeed the activities of the Law Reform Commission in Canada are doing
much to stimulate thoughtful debate, let alone ultimate legal change,
in such areas.

Professor Moskop points out the contention of Robert Veatch, that,
just because a physician has expertise in medical knowledge, it is erroneous to assume that he also has expertise in making value judgments
or moral decisions. Quite rightly Moskop argues that treatment decisions are largely moral decisions or value judgments, and the doctor
therefore cannot shrink from making such judgments even if he/she so
desired. I believe it is perhaps even more erroneous to assume that the
average citizen is more knowledgeable about value judgments than the
physicians. Especially in the medical sphere, the judgments being made
are about the value of a patient's life, and as such, he or she is much
less able to be dispassionate or objective. To phrase it differently,
there are medical moral judgments, and there are non-medical moral
judgments. I would contend that contrary to Veatch's contention, the
doctor must make medical value judgments, but not necessarily in isolation from the patient, the family, or doctors. This is everyday activity for the best physician. I found ironic the situation portrayed in
a recent film regarding the Karen Quinlan case. Although the film may
not be totally accurate, it pointed out that about a year passed while
the courts decided whether Karen's parents were her legal guardians
while she was in a coma, even though she was of legal age. Only after
the courts acted could the parents make the decision as to the potential withdrawal of life-support systems. Many doctors have to make such
a decision several times daily and could not wait for a year for all of
the people in the drama plus a number of legal interpreters to come to
such a decision.

Dr. Roy opens the question of the moral authority of the physician
by dealing directly with the situation of the dying patient. To his
question, "Can professionals be the masters of the art of dying in any
case other than their own?" one can only answer "yes." Whether professionals *should* be the masters of dying in cases other than their own
is more debatable. I find myself agreeing with his terse statement,
"Dying is meant to be an act of life, an act of communication, an act
of integration. Professional skills are meant to serve the achievement
of that act." I tend to feel that my personal bias, is, in fact,

rather widely held. He quite rightly points out that the decision
whether to sustain life, or to refrain from actively intervening during
obvious dying, has far-reaching implications. Uncomfortable as I become in trying to grapple with these matters, I have to acknowledge that
once again this is happening daily at the bedsides of our patients, and
our very own loved ones. The recent public interest in more compassion-
ate professional and social attitudes towards death to me is healthy,
not unexpected. I am particularly pleased that our major religious de-
nominations are courageously trying to deal with these issues openly,
with concern and love, and in this way are trying to make the professed
faith of many of our citizens relevant to the most important aspects of
their lives. I am puzzled by Dr. Roy's comment that, "those who can
successfully define quality of life wield enormous power." Has this
not always been so? That is, those who can define a problem begin immediately to be among those who will have some control over that problem or concern.

Dr. Roy pushes this further, uncomfortably so, and I can only acknowledge the dilemmas. They will become increasingly complex, what
with DNA recombinant genes, cloning potential, and the determination of
sex and sex-linked disease by amniocentesis and fetoscopy early in
pregnancy. Whether humans wish to take the leap toward a sterile eugenic approach to purify the human race seems highly doubtful in light
of Hitler's experiment in that direction four decades ago. Again, I
can only acknowledge the rightness of Dr. Roy's contention that whether
they seek it deliberately, maliciously, or not, those scientists who
continue to develop the technology underlying these potentials, do in
fact wield great power. One quickly thinks, with concern, of the subsequent fate of many of the scientists and service people involved in
the production and delivery of the first atomic bombs. It is my impression that a goodly number subsequently developed significant emotional disease.

One has limits. As Dr. Roy leads me progressively along the path
of larger and larger social issues, I become weary, impatient, irrit-
able, and despairing. I wish to retreat to the bedside, to have to
deal with the moral judgments and value judgments of one other human
being only, the patient of the moment. I willingly accept the responsibilities inherent in that relationship as Professors Moskop and Picard
have outlined them for me. I begin to wish that somehow I did not have
power. That admission acknowledges my recognition that I do have power,
moral authority, and therefore moral responsibility. Dr. Roy ends his

paper with a direct challenge to that kind of responsibility, pointing
out that "real moral authority emerges only when an unrestricted desire
for moral knowledge is matched by equally unrestricted readiness to
achieve consistency between one's doing and one's knowing." Power of
itself doesn't equate with moral authority. Rhetorically he asks, how
do we then "arrive at those higher integrations of human living that
condition the emergence of the higher viewpoints required to match our
power? How can we possibly manage to arrive at a sustained development
of rational self-consciousness, in ourselves and within the community?"
I can only answer--"With great difficulty!"--which is much like trying
to answer the question posed by one man to his friend, "How do two por-
cupines make love?", to which his friend wisely responded, "Carefully--
very carefully."

I agree with Professor Picard that the confidentiality inherent in
the doctor-patient relationship seems in many ways to be breached with
increasing ease. Many national insurance companies have established an
information bank, and in small print advise a prospective client that
the information gained as part of the policy medical examination will be
pooled in that bank unless the client specifically requests in writing
otherwise. Laboratories are compelled by law to report certain diseases. In Alberta that includes mandatory reporting of the finding of
malignant tissue. Within the past couple of years the province of Alberta announced that the records of all patients who have been treated
in an in-patient provincial mental health facility will be put in a computer and thus be available to anyone who can "enter" the computer.
This implies a potential for abuse which did not exist when records were
local to one institution only. Finally, doctors are probably still uncertain as to whether in fact a court of law can demand revelation of
confidential information or not. Professor Picard resolves that un-
certainty yet points out that judges have been reluctant to compel doctors to testify in spite of a legal right to do so. There are many
times of late that doctors feel that *they* are much more concerned about
the confidentiality of the doctor-patient relationship than are patients. Such a viewpoint usually includes a strong and angry conviction that compulsory, universal, medical coverage has contributed a
great deal to this breakdown in the traditional, confidential, doctor-
patient relationship.

Professor Moskop deals with the results of direct public subsidization of health care services at greater length. Interestingly he

says, "In this area of reform, Canada has assumed a clear position of
leadership in North America." I question whom it is that Canada is
leading and where are they all going? Certainly provincial health insurance programs now cover virtually the total population of Canada.
Prepaid medical health insurance programs covered the great majority of
the total population of Canada prior to the federal "medicare" plan being imposed. Most of the major programs at that time were also physi-
cian-founded and well accepted. The Canadian plan, as contrasted to
the English model of the National Health Service, was designed not to
change the structure of medical practice or interfere with the authority of physicians. The programs have in fact done just that. They have
frustrated hospital administrators, created a crisis in the nursing profession, initiated an exodus of physicians to the United States, frustrated physicians, significantly reduced the comparable incomes of physicians when related to the general working population and cost-of-
living indices, and directly influenced many aspects of day-to-day
practice such as choice of tests, frequency of visits, and previously
established referral patterns. Contrary to the implications throughout
the land that Canadian medical costs in total have sky-rocketed, it has
been repeatedly pointed out that, as a percentage of the gross national
product (GNP), Canadian total health care costs have actually fallen in
the last nine years. Justice Emmett Hall himself has noted this fact
and asserted that it should be more widely reported. The May 1980
Reader's Digest has pointed out that, of a number of professions and
occupations, the doctor has suffered the most in regard to an actual
loss of income in the last decade.

Professor Moskop makes specific comments regarding the extension
of benefits of medical care to previosuly underserved groups of citizens, and argues that only social and political action can achieve these
ends. He makes no mention of the "over-served" people. He points out
that, perhaps the Veatch argument regarding the generalization of expertise would hold that physician's medical expertise does not give them
special insight into how health needs of *populations* can best be satisfied. One can equally argue that the expertise of non-medical bureaucrats, medical administrators, politicians, or health consumers doesn't
necessarily give them special insight into how the health needs of populations can best be satisfied either. Further, he suggests that interest in informed consent, the protection of human subjects of medical
research, and the provision of health care for disadvantaged people

does not guarantee their acceptance in everyday medical practice. He
overlooks the fact that these "formal rights" of patients may not necessarily have been in the best interests of patients either. I am not
prepared then to agree completely with him when he states, "I believe
that these reforms are firmly based on fundamental human values of autonomy and dignity, and that reasoned efforts on their behalf should
have our strong support." Cautious support might be a better term.

I am appalled, as I sense is Professor Moskop, with the suggestions
by Illich and Szasz that there be no state support for medicine in any
way. My previous remarks would suggest my disillusionment and disagreement with aspects of the present Canadian "medicare" scheme. This has
to be clearly distinguished from the concept of shared-cost prepaid medical insurance. I firmly believe the vast majority of Canadian physicians strongly support this concept. The great argument is that our
present system is far from perfect; it is too easily exploited, intrudes
on the patient-doctor relationship itself, and negatively influences the
rights, rewards, and dignity of the medical practitioner.

Moskop eloquently refutes Szasz and Illich better than I could.
His subsequent suggestions regarding measures to be taken in the training of new doctors and in the social recognition of physicians to best
foster technical competence, commitment to the welfare of the patient,
and sensitivity to the sick person, are not to be accepted without scrutiny. Certainly incompetent practitioners should be identified and
either barred from practice or made to improve their skills to an acceptable level. This is being done at present. Proposals regarding
limited licensure or mandatory re-licensure are at first glance sensi-
ble. Interestingly, some of the jurisdictions which rushed towards
implementing schemes of this sort some years ago are now quietly trying
to modify or even rescind such programs, as they are proving almost impossible to implement.

I agree with Professor Moskop that moral commitment and sensitivity
can be fostered. To date the data would seem to contradict his contention that the careful selection of prospective physicians for this purpose can be done or is of any predictive value. Perhaps this possibility is hampered by our inability to develop a reliable "empathy index" or
to devise tools which can in fact select individuals who have the capacity to perceive, let alone promote, an acceptable quality of life for
others. I personally propose that once students are selected, on whatever basis, that much more can be done to emphasize the "art of

medicine" not just with potential doctors, but with all other disciplines in the health care team. My observation is that the students coming into these professions are indeed highly motivated, sensitive, and anxious to help their fellow human beings. Regretfully, one observes that after three or four years of training, a lot of such idealism has been culled out or submerged.

Our three speakers have not touched on one of the greatest issues in Canadian medicine today. When he was Minister of Health, the Honourable Marc Lalonde made a noble effort to direct attention towards self-induced illness, i.e., life-style illnesses. Further, the Federal Government has courageously developed and promoted programs attempting to prove that life-style can be influenced positively, and I think that this has been done with considerable success. The Participaction Program and, more recently, the Dialogues on Drinking are having very distinct effects. Consideration of value judgments in medicine must of necessity include situations such as a patient with inappropriately advanced vascular disease, partly due to a chronic heavy smoking habit, who continues to smoke even while recovering from amputation of a limb due to the vascular disease. In the average emergency room the attitude of staff members towards a patient who has deliberately overdosed with ingestion of pills often differs from that towards a middle-aged, overweight, mildly hypertensive, smoking, daily drinking male with an acute heart attack and cardiac arrest. Why? What are we willing to do about it as a consequence? The large sums that have helped promote organ transplants, dialysis programs, banking of human parts, have to be reassessed and moral judgments made because of the limitations on funds. Does our society want to spend huge amounts of money on improving liver transplant techniques or on trying to persuade people to stop abusing alcohol and creating liver problems, let alone widespread social misery, and carnage on the highways? Can the physician obtain some direction regarding moral judgments to be made regarding the individual patient who reflects both the fascinations and the biases of the society in which he lives?

Our speakers have provoked many questions, supplied some answers and given a great deal of information. I remind the thoughtful people at this conference that these are not abstract matters, but are the very fabric of the daily life of the doctor. The speakers have provoked me, a bedside clinician, to acknowledge the power of the health care professions, and to recognize some serious challenges that demand resolution.

THE EMERGENCE OF

MODERN MEDICAL AUTHORITY

THE POLITICAL ECONOMY OF HEALTH IN FRANCE 1770-1830:
THE DEBATE OVER HOSPITAL AND HOME CARE AND
IMAGES OF THE WORKING-CLASS FAMILY*

HARVEY MITCHELL

The controversy over the respective merits of hospital and home
care for the working-class between the 1770s and 1830s in France raises
a number of provocative questions and vexing problems that continue to
find an echo among laymen, people in the medical professions, and
scholars. My indirect purpose in this study is to consider the degree
to which Michel Foucault's[1] depiction of the medicalization of France is
accurate. My chief purpose is to see how medical men became one of the
major groups to dominate thought and practice on these matters before,
but unmistakably after, the Revolution.[2] I will show how they tried to
come to terms with, and to exercise constraints over, shifting, growing,
not easily definable groups of workers, who inspired as much fear as
compassion: artisans with skills that were variously esteemed; the
laboring poor of town and city who plied a bewildering number of trades
and services, the most primitive of which depended on the use of unaided
muscle power; and workers in the newer manufacturing establishments
where they performed simple, but often dangerous, machine operations.
All of them contributed to the formation of the heterogeneous working-
class of the nineteenth century.

The conscious decision of medical men to take an active role in
determining the future of this class may perhaps best be understood
within the context of an emergent political economy. The will to shape,
direct, and dominate was older, to be sure, but economic growth and the
advocates of a science of political economy, especially during the latter part of the period under survey, gave a new urgency to medical
claims. The halo of enlightened science surrounded and helped to give a
certain sanctity to their endeavours. By contrast with the present-day
loss of absolute confidence in science and scientific activity, which

*I wish to thank the Social Sciences and Humanities Research Coun-
cil of Canada for a grant which made the research for this paper possible.

originates partly in the self-doubt of some scientists, the end of the
eighteenth and the beginning of the nineteenth century were truly marked
by an incredible sense of imminent material, scientific, and in some
minds, too, of moral, achievement.[3] But the implicit promises of medical activity often threatened, it must be added, to dissolve altogether,
not because medical men doubted their high purpose, which little could
disturb, but because they were still exploring the relationship of medicine to science, and were not at all certain that their interventions
were making a great enough impact on the health of the population. As
practical men--hence not only as "pure" theorists or scholars--they were
sensitive to the world around them, could not be oblivious to the social functions of medicine, and readily assumed some of its burdens,
but they were largely not aware of the extent to which their own work
as practitioners and as theorists was shaped by the productive process.
Hence their efforts to extend their therapeutic effectiveness and to improve their professional status, both of which entailed the development
of a series of linked disciplinary microstructures, could not be smooth.
While they cast themselves in the role of humane and moral guides, ac-
tuated only by the most untarnished of motives, they were not always
seen as they saw themselves. Since their language and their concerns
were not primarily attuned to the vocabulary which expressed the thinking of others--entrepreneurs, manufacturers, and property-owners--whose
relationship to the productive process was more direct, their ambiguous
position in society was thereby revealed, as was their vulnerability.

My paper will look at the arguments for and against hospital and
home care. The voices most affected will not be excluded: the poor,
the deviant, the marginal, the old, and the sick, who cannot always be
easily distinguished from the productive and physically able, hence com-
paratively independent, members of the working-class. My interpretation
will rely heavily on an assessment of the dominant groups, because that
is my chief purpose, and also because decoding the wishes of the second
is beyond my reach. Speculation will sometimes have to substitute for
empirical data. For the same reasons, it will be the images, for the
most part, not the self-images of the working-class family, that I shall
try to recapture. My concern rests on, and owes much of its energy
from, the theme of power and authority in medical care. I take this to
mean, within the confines of my study, first, how and why they came to
be used to enhance some values and deny others; second, an obligation to
keep in mind that such procedures tend to improve the lives of some more

readily than others; and, third, adequate acknowledgment of the emotional and intellectual conflicts that were part of the process.

   Medical discussion of the forms of care stemmed from the medical
philosophy of the period. It was concerned with what I should like to
call a field of multiple social, environmental, and biological forces
within which human beings were said to move from a state of health to a
state of disease and back again. Insofar as the locus of medical care
was seen as helping to determine the movement from a condition of disease to one of health, the preference for one form of care over the
other should have logically rested on ideas and practices which were as
much a part of the social as of the medical realm. Nevertheless, medical men did not always keep the interaction of the two realms in mind,
and often reified[4] notions of health and disease, as if they existed
outside the social realm altogether. It is not always easy to know when
this was being done, but it was more evident in the curative rather than
the preventive aspects of medicine. A similar hazard lay in wait for
others--politicians, public administrators, philanthropists--who shared
the responsibility for imposing authority on the activities of working-
class families. In this process, they showed themselves capable of creating totally unreal demands upon them by manufacturing the symbols of a
new kind of family, responsible and temperate, yet deferential and submissive. When medical men combined both tendencies in their own thought
and practice, the implications could be extraordinarily revealing. One
of these, for a time, was to place excessive stress on the desirability
of a static, stable, and unchanging society. By the end of the first
third of the nineteenth century, so confining a goal could no longer be
pressed so convincingly or so vehemently. By then, medical men had
erected an ideology, long in the making, which tended to conflate medical and economic advance, and made them in many respects mutually dependent.

I

Hospital and Home Care

   In one important respect, the debate over hospital and home care
arose from an acutely perceived need to clarify the purposes of poor and
medical relief. This complex structure of social assistance could no
longer easily endure the pressures of a changing economy that appeared
to be increasing the numbers of people living as unproductive members of

society. Of course, the issues could not be totally visible to those
caught up in the controversy. There was a greater sensitivity to, and
irritation with, the apparently unending demands made on society by both
its undesirable and unfortunate groups than there was of the economy's
capacity to deal with, and society's responsibility for, them. Custod-
ial care evolved over some centuries to the point where the word "hospital" had come to mean the provision of a continuum of overlapping
forms of care and relief for several, if not all, groups of people in
acute need of resources for survival, or who existed chronically on the
boundaries of want. What was seen to be at stake in the allocation and
varying uses of hospital spaces, as well as in determining an alternative to them, was the need to interrupt that continuum, so that discrete
functions and precise goals could be achieved in a rational, uniform,
and regular way. At the end of the eighteenth century, the future status of the hospital as an institution for the sick requiring treatment
and expecting care and cure, was undeniably changing, but it remained
far from certain.[5]

What is surprising is that the hospital survived at all. The cres-
cendos of criticism and the expressions of undisguised contempt for the
distance between its ostensible goals and its actual practices were of
such a magnitude that it promised to be one of the more obvious casual-
ties of the Revolutionary period. Instead the hospital was given a new
lease on life. In time, ironically, it came to be valued as having the
capacity to restore people to health. But before the leap to that re-
assessment of its functions was made, before it was seen in that light,
it was thought to be actually producing disease and killing people.
This conviction was never fully eradicated from the minds even of those
who favored its retention in its newer form.

There are several parts to this problem. The most intractable of
them remains how and why members of the medical profession enforced
their "scientific" claims in the hospital setting at a time when there
was no clear evidence that medicine possessed clear and compelling superiority in its theoretical understanding of and practical approach to
illness. The second, in light of this, is how and why the political
authorities perceived and accepted those claims. An important additional element in it were the provisions for home medical care, which had
always been part of the structure of social assistance, but which, like
the facilities in the hospital, were being re-evaluated. The thought
and action evoked by these problems were not lacking in ambiguities of

a singularly high order, not the least of which were those surrounding
the "freedom" associated with home care, and its loss which was seen as
a consequence of hospitalization.

Ambivalence, doubt, and self-questioning alternated with clarity of
intention, evidence that seemed to support it, and confidence in the results of cumulative inquiry. Medical men shared with other critics of
the old regime hospital structure a revulsion for its failings, and continued to express it without interruption after 1789 as well. Some of
them would not flinch from nor deny the high rates of morbidity and mortality in the hospitals, such as the hôtels-Dieu which were exclusively
devoted to medical functions, even if they did not openly indulge in the
lugubrious tones of a lawyer who called for the suppression of the
Hôtel-Dieu on the ground that it was hardly an appropriate place for the
recovery of health. It was, in fact, he said, "a veritable living se-
pulcher."[6] Because of the great stress they were placing on environmental sources of disease, of which the hospital was one, they were also
likely to agree with Delecloy, a politician during the period of the
Directory, who compared Paris, a "city of smoke and filth, of luxury and
misery," to a "great hospital...with its collection of all the human
vices and infirmities...corruption and indigence...."[7] Like other public buildings--but more acutely and uniquely so--the hospital was
thought to be an active source of pollution, because of its diseased
population, and at the same time, a passive receptor of a polluted atmosphere, due to its faulty topographical siting and its non-functional,
monumental architecture. Much of medical thinking on these matters had
been telescoped conveniently in the massive study of Paris's hospitals
by the surgeon Tenon, completed just before the Revolution.[8] That survey, together with the Academy of Sciences' recommendation to construct
four new hospitals in Paris, embodying Tenon's principles of sound construction and therapy, accorded recognition and enormous prestige of an
unprecedented kind to physicians.[9]

Ambiguities of another kind permeated the supposed wishes of the
poor. We know of them principally from the observations of doctors and
other members of the dominant social class. Contrary, however, to what
one of the oldest studies on poor relief in France has enshrined as an
unchallengeable truth,[10] it is difficult to conclude on the basis of the
evidence, which Bloch himself addresses, that the poor universally rejected the hospital and preferred to have their illnesses cared for at
home. Doctors reported, as did the *cahiers de doléances*, a range of

attitudes.[11] In some cases, there was a marked distaste for hospitals
as "gateways to death."[12] In the view of others, the poor were being
denied medical attention because of the monopolization of hospital beds
by the military, a problem that was to become acute during the Revolutionary wars. Masters were said in other instances to have gained
favored and special hospital admission for their servants in exchange
for payment, or because of the terms of particular endowments, thus
blocking permanently what were deemed to be the even older and more legitimate obligations to the poor. Caution is needed in weighing these
grievances and preferences. Both doctors and the drafters of the *cahiers* were capable of distorting the expectations of the poor by super-
imposing their own upon them. There were medical men whose dismay and
indignation at the absence of hospital facilities for the poor was
grounded in an older paternalistic ideology. They continued to express
the wish that the hospital be restored to its traditional functions.
For them that was more important than its clinical promise. As for the
grievances embodied in the *cahiers*, we can explain the wish for expanded
hospital service at government expense as a means for the more favored
sections of the community to be relieved from the burden of direct care
based on charitable donations and local taxes. But the picture is far
from clear.

What we have come face to face with is the insoluble problem of
assessing the expectations of the poor directly. Studies that have used
various methods to penetrate popular consciousness would seem to suggest
that most of the poor, outside the great cities and smaller towns, were
denied the choice, or, to the great dismay of surgeons, apothecaries,
and doctors, simply lacked the capacity or the will to make what were
considered to be "rational" decisions affecting their health.[13] Hospital or home care for most of the population of France would have been an
innovation of truly radical proportions. When it was enshrined as a
principle by the Constituent Assembly,[14] with much greater stress placed
on home care, the dual system envisioned owed much of its substance to
the discussions that had started at least in the 1770s.

The poor knew enough about the great overpopulated hospitals, like
the Paris Hôtel-Dieu, to think of them as a last resort, as institutions
in which they were likely to be callously neglected or in which they
would not survive. That assumption, according to Tenon, was fully justified. The mortality rate was conservatively estimated at about twenty-two per cent.[15] It gains verification from a carefully argued

analysis, which appeared in 1790, of hospital mortality statistics by
Dr. François Doublet who, in the years between 1779 and 1783, had been
a physician at the hospice de Charité in St. Sulpice, the most heavily
populated parish in the city. The Charité was founded as a model institution a year before Doublet's appointment, and was expected to provide
data on the proper functioning of a hospital, including the various
sources of mortality. As far as possible, Doublet used comparative
hospital statistics, including figures from the Paris Hôtel-Dieu, the
Edinburgh Hospital (cited in the Academy's reports), and the hôtel-Dieu
at Nimes. His report carries much authority. He recognized that mortality rates were not simply a function of internal administration,
quality of treatment, building standards, and funding. Indeed, improvements in all of these would have, he asserted, negligible effect
on mortality rates if other less obvious variables were not altered. As
Doublet put it, somewhat euphemistically, existing hospitals were places
in which the greatest proportion of illnesses were not "accessible to
the power of medicine." They were instead institutions that managed
death, because their patients were "marked by death before their admission." In fact, the hospitals were emblematic of the entire community's disease structure, and because of this mortality rates could only
be identical with those of a city or of society as a whole. He completed his analysis by considering the contribution of such variables as
age, sex, and civilian/military distribution to the overall mortality
rates. [16]

Doublet was arguing that the hospital could no longer bear the
burden of caring for the undifferentiated mass of the sick and of the
poor, and that if the stigma which it carried were removed, it could
proceed to carry out its remedial work with success. Thus the technical
and medical reorganization of the hospital would deal much more effectively with disease. The public authorities, lay and medical, would decide the nature of the population's distribution within the hospital
structure, ensuring the provision of a series of marked-off spaces to
meet specific and "unrelated" needs. Medical men argued that objecti-
fication and diagnosis of illness as disease in the hospital, populated
by the poor and needy, was essential to the advancement of medicine.
Thus the poor were seen chiefly as bearers of disease, while doctors
saw themselves as bearers of an improved semiotics and nosology. [17]

This increasingly self-conscious expectation of medical men is evident in their arguments for the hospital as a therapeutic centre, a

teaching institution, and a scientific observing post. In addition,
the information collected by the Société Royale de Médecine, which was
revealing the extent and limitations of orthodox medical practices, the
practices of competing systems of healing, and the condition of the human and animal populations, unquestionably reduced medical hesitations,
but did not remove them.[18] There were still enormous resistances and
barriers, not the least of which were physicians' own responses to the
two faces of medicine, the prophylactic and the curative, and the complex ways in which the two were related and interacted. Certainly physicians wished to stretch out their hands to encompass both. Their
writings were transparent celebrations of their superior culture, dedi-
cation, and potential benefactions to suffering humanity.[19] Men like
Vicq d'Azyr, Cabanis, Flandrin, Fourcroy, Moreau de la Sarthe, and
others shared the common vocabulary of enlightened medical philosophy
and experience in hospital work, administrative posts, and in the larger
community. During the Revolution, some of them even participated in
political life as elected deputies. These aspects of their thought and
activities are not in dispute, but if their claims and those of their
successors in the next generation established their authority in the
medical domain, their success was partial, only a beginning, and, most
important, rested on a mixture of rather slender achievements, grandiose
ambitions, and some rather unjustified optimism. It is easy, however,
to detect the split in their thinking, between their faith in medical
change and the state of the art itself. Their acknowledgment of how
much they still had to know was a confession of how little they knew.
They directed themselves to the future to give some of their pretentions
credence in the present. So determined were they to establish a "research programme" through observation in a clinical setting, that we can
understand some of the grounds for the hospital's survival.[20]

The paradox is that most of them endorsed home care for most of the
working population. Superficially, their position, which was supported
by most sections of educated lay opinion, seems incontrovertibly per-
suasive and rational. For one, the crowded and overtaxed structure of
institutionalized care appeared in danger of collapse, even if after its
reorganization the sick poor were forced to seek medical care in it.
The goal was, at this level of the argument, to reduce both the hospital population and hospital costs, and this could be done by reserving
its facilities rigorously and uniquely for those totally deprived of
family support, as well as for those with intractable or unusual medical

problems. In addition, for the vast numbers of the urban and rural
poor of France, medical care dispensed in a family and neighborhood
setting was much the superior form of treatment, and the preference,
they argued, of the poor themselves. Disease, as Foucault phrased it,
would be captured in "a double system of observation," in the family,
which was "the natural locus of disease," and in the hospital, which
duplicated, "like a microcosm, the specific configuration of the pathological world."[21] Thus both the social and medical needs of the population would be met.

        Doctors did indeed refer to the family as the natural locus of dis-
ease, but some, like Chambon de Montaux, in the late 1780s, were convinced that it was precisely for this reason that patients should be removed from its baneful environmental and social influences if they were
to benefit from medical intervention.[22] Disease would be conquered
through observation in the hospital, if anywhere. In a sense, then,
this generation of doctors was claiming the necessity of devoting the
largest part of their energies to the remedial side of medicine, and
they left it to be implied--because they did not openly disavow or were
as yet unable to discuss a future role for themselves in broader schemes
of preventive medicine, including legal medicine--that the real future
of medicine lay with the first rather than the second. Were these beliefs shared by those who advocated home care? Much more thought must
be given to the prevailing ideology that tended to enshrine it as the
ideal, for what it was purported to achieve and its relationship to the
environment in which the population lived and worked have not been satisfactorily investigated. To this problem I shall return later.

        Home care was envisioned as simple and inexpensive, and above all
as responsive to the emotional, economic, and social needs of working-
class families. It would ideally flourish in a decentralized system
and directly involve the members of the community who would be given an
opportunity to express and expand their sense of unity with and compassion for the afflicted. By its very nature, it would resist the deper-
sonalized bureaucracy of the state and of the hospital which was the
state in microcosm. As the Comité de mendicité declared in their fourth
report, it would enhance personal pride, initiative, and independence.
The state would thus be prevented from becoming the sole means of support for the needy individual.[23] Earlier Chambon appeared to get over
the difficulty of endowing the state with such powers by speaking of a
free contract between the rich and the poor through the intermediary of

the hospital and its privileged practitioners, the physicians. According to him, it would facilitate an equitable exchange between the rich whose taxes would maintain it, and the poor who would be given free care in it, their only obligation being the subjection of their bodies to medical investigation. Thus the reciprocal needs of both classes in society would be served.[24] Chambon was a frank advocate of a system that would turn its back, for all practical purposes, on exploring the connections between economic life, social institutions, and disease. The poor, he seemed to be saying, had no choice but to take their chances in the world of labor. When they fell ill, as was inevitable they would, however, not be abandoned.

Self-reliance cultivated through home care, and the development within the working-class family of a stricter sense of mutual obligation and planning, were ideas which, from their inception, were not free from vestiges of paternalism and deference. In the cold language of Dupont de Nemours, the poor were caught in a world in which he urged them to make their own way by becoming, as far as possible, prudential, providing for their needs in times of illness. But he did not envisage economic prudence as an instrument by means of which social class could be breached. Neither under the old regime, nor later when he was a Napoleonic official and active in philanthropic works, did Dupont see any problem in reconciling his aphorism, "God helps those who help themselves," with minimal state assistance and charitable works.[25] Perhaps his physiocratic principles, which did not accord productive value to non-agricultural workers, but extended maximum value to landed proprietors and self-sufficient peasants, prevented him from supporting a programme exclusively devoted to home care. Hence the freedom which a system of home care was supposed to promote seems as severely restricted as Chambon's putative freedom mediated metaphorically through a hospital contract, reconciling the interests of rich and poor.

For the political authorities, especially the policing officials in great cities like Paris, the "good" worker was fervent in and dedicated to his work, loyal to his master, and moving through time within the various hierarchies of different groups of skilled workers. Louis-Sébastien Mercier's alarm that orderly work routines were vanishing, provoking a whirlpool of social chaos, was shared by others in all ranks and conditions within the privileged community, even if they lacked his expressive powers. He deplored the threats to a social and legal structure in which domestic servants had known their place. His conviction

that every domestic servant in Paris was both a source of evil and cor-
ruption and a loss to the agrarian resources of the country doubtless
comes from his acquaintance with physiocratic principles. He contrasted
the armies of domestic servants favorably, however, with the seditious,
mutinous, totally public way of life of the poor in the working-class
faubourg Saint-Marcel, in lodging houses, where whole families crowded
together in one room.[26]   For his contemporary, Montyon, who poured out
his zeal in vast collections of social statistics, the urban workers, on
the other hand, were inherently dangerous, whether they were marginal or
skilled, with or without a family, since the havoc caused by unemployment and disease reduced them all to the same level and created chronic
instability.[27]

     Eligibility for domiciliary care meant, in the first instance, to
be legally domiciled, and crucially, in time of sickness, with the members of one's family. The domicile was a measure, in bourgeois eyes, of
self-identity, identification, fixity, regularity, dependability--the
very opposite of rootlessness and vagabondage.[28] This distinction lay
at the root of the two kinds of care. To be non-domiciled meant quite
automatically to lack any of the resources required to cultivate the
habits of self-help. Without them, care given in the home was a contradiction in terms. If the ideal was the development of family values
within a fixed setting, it was conceived--and it continued to be seen in
this way for some time in the future--as being only distantly realizable
for large numbers of the poor, if at all. The aim was to increase the
pool of the responsible members of the poor, or, to use the older term,
the deserving sections of this large and heterogeneous class which required all the legal ingenuity of the old régime lawyers and policing
authorities to find proper places for them. What the Revolution tried
to achieve in the realm of medical and other forms of assistance was to
find local roots for the infirm, the old, and the sick in the family and
parish, to maximize mutual forms of aid, and, when that was not possible,
to institutionalize the others. The purpose of home care was to keep an
eye on, to know at all times who constituted the family, who lived in
the section, parish, district, etc., and thus to acquire the information
to exercise effective control and impose rigorous cost-accounting procedures. The English sytem of poor relief was increasingly but not universally adduced--Cabanis was a dissenting voice--as an example of the
virtues of locally controlled assistance.[29] This amounted to fixing the
poor in a known location, to immobilizing them.

Barère, one of the more moderate members of the Committee of Public Safety, had almost as much faith in the family to exercise its re-
cuperative power on the sick, as he had contempt for the hospitals
which he believed would lose their claim for privileged status in society as quickly as charity encouraged by obscurantist religion would
lose its rationale. Enormously underestimating the number of the in-
digent--his figure was five per cent of the total population--he spoke
in ringing tones of the family as generative of human dignity, economic
prudence, and civic pride, all of which were endangered and depleted in
the hospital at the hands of the very men and women who had been appointed to their posts to assist those in need. He urged the Convention to remove the words charity and hospitals from the sacred vocabulary of the Republic.[30]

They were not expunged. Developments after Thermidor were in
sharp contrast with the more radical phases of the Convention, and
even with the earlier work of the Constituent Assembly. When Dr.
Thouret, one of the two medical members of the Comité de Mendicité of
1789-1791 invoked Adam Smith's *Wealth of Nations*, he did so not to favor a market economy, but rather to support the position that parish-
based assistance was too costly, wasteful, and inhumane. He argued
that the poor were the total responsibility of the state and that control over them was needed to prevent them from becoming the victims of
decisions made locally and perhaps capriciously.[31] But neither the
Comité nor its successors in the more radical régimes that followed
ever opposed the concept of domiciliary care. The principle was maintained even after the dismantling of the Convention's laws, including
the law of March 19, 1793, which had promised work for all, the end of
charity, and assistance for those who had met all the tests of need,
and, of course, Barère's law of 22 floréal an II (May 11, 1794) nation-
alizing hospital property. Delecloy's report of 12 vendémiaire an IV
(October 1795) successfully challenged the principles of centralized
help, and the hospitals were restored to the control of the municipalities.[32] There would thenceforth be no fiscal charge on the state.
Delaporte, for example, in July 1796 in the Conseil des Cinq-Cents,
demonstrated his total commitment to locally administered assistance on
the English model and argued that real costs had not really risen. If
the poor congregated more heavily in some communes than in others, it
was due to the relative wealth and opportunities that were to be found
there, not because the system was breaking down, as its critics claimed

both in England and in France.[33] Two years later, he was able apparently to conclude that there were links between the new legislation,
which he had predicted would put an end to debauchery and family irre-
sponsibility,[34] and the great change wrought by the earlier destruc-
tion of the guilds, the laborer's freedom to work wherever he chose,
a fair standard of living, a strengthened family, and savings to tide
them over when illness struck.[35]

In its summary of its philosophy and in its proposals, the Directory in 1798 openly acknowledged what was in the minds of many who had
been participating in the debate for such a long time. Contradictory
laws had thrown hospital administrators into confusion and anxiety, the
Directors said. The problem had started with the ill-advised attempts
of the Constituent Assembly to think of:

> the poor classes as the exclusive responsibility
> of the government alone; they are more particularly
> the responsibility of those who have delivered them
> to heavy work, and have, as it were, created pover-
> ty. It is therefore a duty for the well-to-do
> classes to care for the poor classes who have pro-
> cured their riches or goods for them; it is in the
> distinction made between the duties that are the
> government's and those that are the individual's
> that one must seek the theory of public assistance.
>   A government that would announce that it would
> on its own grant complete assistance to all the
> poor, and in every one of life's stages, would as-
> sume an enormous burden. It would destroy industry;
> it would encourage lack of concern in the rich, and
> it would crush private charity which is the motivating
> force behind sociability.[36]

The minister of the Interior, Letourneux, in his report to the Directory, which acted on his recommendations in its message to the Conseil
des Cinq-Cents, supported the English structure of local assistance,
and indirectly endorsed, so it seems, Smith's principle of self-interest, by declaring that "the dangers and numbers of the poor (would)
diminish immediately, when personal and general interests were brought
into conflict." This convoluted endorsement of Smith's theories was
predicated on a rejection of the theory that the general interest could
be sought intentionally by the government's exclusive solicitude for
the poor. Again the expected economies from an expanded system of
domiciliary care and a severely reduced hospital establishment were
pressed home.[37]

The Directors were caught, as was Letourneux, between the older
principles of charity, which they tended to idealize, the more innovative propositions favoring the supremacy of self-interest, and the

even more candid allusion to the causes of poverty. In successive
months, reporting for the Conseil des Cinq-Cents' commission on hospitals, Jouenne criticized domiciliary care as a totally unrealistic
system for "that class of useful citizens who have no domicile, for
those artisans in all occupations who work in workshops, in manufactor-
ies, for those men who lodge chiefly in inns, for domestic servants of
both sexes, for those employed in rural work, all of whom in their
infirmities have no other resources than the hospices where they can be
treated." He resisted the project to cut down the number of hospitals,
and recognized that the economic realities were such as to preclude
such a heavy commitment to home care.[38]

The theory of political economy which was emerging from the debates embraced a number of competing positions. It is not part of my
purpose to consider that part of the debate which centred on the merits
of adopting a system of public bids for hospital purchase of supplies,
except to note that deputies such as Delecloy and Porcher, who defended
many of the points in the Directory's programme, pointed out the in-
compatibility between profits and morality, contracts and philanthro-
py.[39] Jouenne's allusions of the year before to the actual housing of
workers were, however, deliberately ignored, and the principle of home
care was implicitly reaffirmed, when it was not directly praised.
Delecloy's aversion, as he labelled them, for all those "eloquently
written, but ridiculous and absurd systems" which had demolished "those
sacred asylums of relief, those majestic retreats..." was a reference
to the radical legislation of a few years before. Individual philan-
thropy would, he predicted, be restored, and private compassion re-
warded.[40]

When the legislators during the period of the Directory and later
when the administrators of domiciliary and hospital care in the Paris
region expressed their dismay at and could not restrain their impatience[41] with a social and medical problem that resisted all their
good intentions and their seemingly rational programmes, it was likely
due to their uncertain blending of two incompatible elements in a
hybridized political economy. Paternalism, apprehension, and prudence
stood like watchdogs blocking entry through the portals of a political
economy of "free" and mobile labor. Foundations for what may be
called the technologies of power and authority, with the additional
purpose of mitigating the principles and practices of a "free" labor
market, were consequently laid down by the deputies. Medical men

gained political support for their hospital scheme by appealing to a
vision which rested more on a promise of future than actual medical advances. The hospital survived, and indeed flourished in the era of
clinical medicine, not because it radically and dramatically reversed
mortality rates or produced a cumulative record of cures, although this
remained the constant aim of medicine. Rather, for the political authorities, it was meant to serve the double purpose of dealing with an
irreducible proportion of the poor and needy, who could find no other
refuge, and as a deterrent to such workers who were expected to take
seriously the task of self-improvement in the home, where a new generation of laboring people was seen, as it were, emerging from the bosom
of the family as responsible members of a future "free" labor force.
The preservation of the family as a viable reproductive and productive
unit, with its affective ties strengthened and its links of sociability
and mutuality in the neighborhood strengthened, was the fanciful side
of a hard-headed policy. The latter was really pledged to a theory of
human nature that called on disciplinary agents to arouse and support
supposed universal human instincts of sympathy and sentiment. The
"true" nature of the worker would be given every opportunity to flourish, but the proper environment for him, as well as the proper sphere
of medicine, were still part of the future.[42]

II

Mutual Aid Societies and Occupational Medicine

Two preferred policies were conceived as marking the passage from
the older to the newer forms of assistance and public health. Each
complemented the other. Together they may be seen as a composite social and biological prescription for health, and as the most acceptable
form of prophylaxis. The first of these, the mutual aid societies, de-
nuded of their original political goals, constituted the exact antithe-
sis of working-class-initiated schemes of self-realization and self-
definition, which had been such an unwelcome feature of the more radical phase of the Revolution. These mutual aid, benefit, friendly, or
burial societies were established as early as the 1780s and grew in
number in the early years of the nineteenth century. With their membership from the world of the skilled trades, this élite of the working
class was mainly literate and highly conscious of guild traditions. It
was to them that sponsors of savings banks appealed, as in the case of
André-Jean de la Rocque's *Société bienfaisante*, which hoped to attract

modest savings from skilled workers. De la Rocque, author of two such
projects, proposed an establishment which would bring together "the
skilled worker and the capitalist and increase the wealth of both by
investing the money of the second through the work and industry of the
first."[43] The societies were in the main self-actuating, mixing a
sense of solidarity with prudent militance. In the years following the
passage of the Chapelier Law of 1791, which emasculated the societies
and made strikes illegal, the idea of working-class mutual aid came increasingly to fall under the watchful eye of philanthropists whose
thinking was often indistinguishable from the paternalistic attitudes
of pre-Revolutionary times.[44] In 1803, Pastoret, conservative veteran
of Revolutionary assemblies, dignitary of the Napoleonic régime, and
president of the Paris-based *Société philanthropique*, urged workers to
follow the lead taken by the employees of the Réveillon paper factory,
who, under Messrs. Jacquemart and Bénard, continued to support on their
own, with no matching contributions, a benefit fund in order, as it was
said, to ensure that "illnesses are not embittered by despair" and to
promise an old age which is "only the calm evening of a day passed in
work."[45] There is an obvious connection between the ideology of home
medical care, the societies, and the encouragement given them by people
such as Dupont de Nemours, who saw them as enabling workers to look after themselves through their savings in times of unemployment.[46]

According to a government report, probably dating from 1806, there
were some sixty-four such societies in Paris with an average membership
of eighty, some confined to one trade, others with a heterogeneous occupational membership, and two of which were exclusively made up of
women. Two features of these organizations are very much worth noting.
The first point has already been made: the societies were the preserve
principally of the most economically favored members of the working
class. High entrance fees and high minimum annual contributions saw to
that. The second is that, whatever the larger aims of the societies
were, including the degree to which they challenged their employers or
authority in general--a matter that demands research--they were seen by
officials of the state, and also by private individuals who took an active part in promoting the workers' groups, as the bulwark of "order,
economy, and good morals in their families."[47] At least during the
Napoleonic period, they were thought to be no threat to social peace.
They were so timid, it was said, that the slightest suggestion of police surveillance would see to their voluntary disbandment.[48]

Submissiveness suffused the declarations of an *Association de bien-faisance mutuelle*, founded in 1809, and still going strong ten years later under the Restoration. With a membership overwhelmingly of printers, it wished, it proclaimed, to maintain social harmony and stability and to confine hospital care, which it believed was less desirable, exclusively for workers in the least lucrative trades. As for themselves, their society would, in time of illness and old age, be a source of support when the worker was no longer able to "establish a perfect balance between his wages and his expenses."[49] The nine free schools in the faubourg Saint-Germain, which had been established by a private lay organization, set out as one of the keys to a successful curriculum for the children of the poor the obligation to teach them to "calculate their small expenses, to make them appreciate the advantages of order, work, and good behavior, to make of them, in a word, workers; more intelligent servants than those who have learned nothing; soldiers able to achieve the ranks they [had within themselves] the power to deserve..." "As for women, [it was necessary] to make them good workers, good housekeepers, useful to their husbands, and nothing more."[50]

One of the members of the younger generation of Idéologues, Joseph-Marie de Gérando, devoted much of his thought and energies during and after the Restoration to the problems of identifying the roots of indigence, but his claims on our attention lie in his self-proclaimed wish to penetrate, as it were, the mentality of working-class people, so as to gain the right to direct them towards a larger control over their lives. Earlier, during the Napoleonic period, he had served on a government commission to look into how the operations of the home care program could be improved. In publishing the first edition of *Le Visiteur du pauvre* in 1820--it went through several editions--de Gérando declared it would be a prelude to a large-scale comparative European study on public assistance. He rejected all notions of economic and social equality, and asserted his belief in the moral foundations uniting rich and poor, which were superior to a morality based exclusively on work. If work, commerce, the sciences, and the arts ruled the universe, then human order and society would amount to nothing but a species of "industrial egoism." With these prefatory remarks, de Gérando devoted the rest of his guide book to seeking out the "self-inflicted" causes of poverty. This, he believed, was a necessary prologue to determining the legitimate beneficiaries of assistance and ensuring the isolation of those incorrigible poor who would not or

should not be helped. De Gérando helped to set the tone for the gradual "professionalization" of agencies ready to intervene in the lives of
working-class people.[51]

Even after 1830, the paternalistic impulses, which were very much
a part of the philanthropic Social Catholic credo as well, and were exemplified in the activities of men like the vicomte de Villeneuve-
Bargemont, remained strong.[52] New economic developments undermining the
foundations of artisanal production, so much of which continued to rest
on the pre-industrial family economy, remained fragmentary and dispersed. The features of the older economy were, to be sure, beginning
to blur a bit, and the features of the new were becoming more discernible, but a factory labor force was far from having established itself
as the dominant form of production throughout France. Indeed the an-
tagonism expressed in philanthropic circles, especially among the Social
Catholics, towards the factory system of labor as a crucible of immorality and as a source of oppression of the weak, often by the weak
themselves, was the very rationale for their efforts to restore family
values. An equally powerful conviction among artisans and other skilled
workers in their capacity to improve their self-image persisted, even
two years after the 1848 Revolution. One of the leading working-class
newspapers, *l'Atelier*, announced its goal in its final issue:

> To react against certain immoral and extravagant
> ideas which used to have currency in our class;--
> To develop among workers the belief in their value
> as producers and of their dignity as citizens; to
> teach them to have more confidence in their own
> powers, to rely increasingly on themselves, and
> less on that deceptive providence that one calls
> the state;--To urge workers unceasingly to seek
> the successive conquest of their instruments of
> work through free and voluntary association;--In
> every case, to have the moral interest prevail
> over the material.[53]

The point to be made is that, well beyond the first decades of the
nineteenth century, a "free" factory labor force was only in the making
in France, and that its advent was, for the most zealous defenders of
paternalistic attitudes, not particularly welcome, since they perceived
it as destructive of an older and superior morality and the voluntary
social institutions that supported it. If these were to be preserved,
if destitution and poverty were to be maintained within manageable
bounds, and if the roots of social peace were to be kept in a healthy
state, the principles of discipline and self-discipline had to be embodied in law. Economic calculation and the profit motive cannot by

themselves account for the development of an ideology of, and a set of strategies leading to, self-improvement. "Fear," as Theodor Adorno has suggested, "constitutes a more crucial subjective motive of objective rationality."[54] In the case before us, fear activated those who exercised power, and it was also seen as activating those upon whom that power would be imposed. The compulsion to use power found much of its legitimacy from the creation of standards of "normal" modes of behavior and some sense or presentiment of how the worst features of "human nature" could perhaps be kept in check or even eradicated. The release of volcanic popular energy was hardly unknown, and the memory of revolutionary activity had burned deeply. Without proper training, the working-class was too dangerous a force to be released in a "free" market. Such a market was simply unthinkable. It would not bind up society; it would promote instead the dissolution of a fragile one.

Medical men, thereby complementing the exertions of the philanthropists, turned their attention to the more apparent consequences of economic and social alterations in the natural environment. As we know, the study of environmental influence on the human constitution has a venerable history in medical thought and practice.[55] It assumed new importance in the eighteenth and nineteenth centuries as a result of a fresh consciousness of the need to combat epidemic, endemic, and epizootic disease. Further study rested on a combined prophylactic and curative strategy. The balance between the two began to shift towards the first in the growing concern to regulate standards for working-class housing and to introduce a series of public hygiene measures, such as an improved water supply, a sewage system, garbage disposal, and clean streets. Such a policy would break, it was confidently expected, the links between poverty and disease. Thinking of this sort was in part an extension of the arguments for home medical care. How much more effective it could be in an unpolluted environment. If more were done to promote both private and public hygiene, the more likely would many diseases begin to disappear. By some powerful mental alchemy, the physician-hygienists-politicians-administrators, like those who were active in the silk industry centre of Lyon in the first decades of the nineteenth century,[56] and in many of the other principal cities of France, believed that, by giving priority to housing, public health improvements, and hospital hygiene, municipal governments would succeed in filtering out many of the more gratuitous forms of disease, leaving behind a fresh precipitate of hygienic morality. Poverty could assume

a disinfected image and the working-class would become less dangerous.
Here the limits to the policy priorities in this general preventive
strategy emerges clearly. The preferred forms of prophylaxis remained
focused on an analysis of the poor, not on the economic system that produced poverty.

At the same time, occupational hazards and diseases could not escape the attention of the medical men. The prolonged examination of men
and women in the workplace would be bound to unearth unsuspected questions and raise alternative approaches to prevailing notions of health
and disease. A journal which was published by a group of doctors and,
for a brief time, jointly with men of letters, from the mid-twenties to
1829, the year before the Revolution of 1830, seemed to register, by
its very change of names in a brief period, an awareness of the growing
importance of the newer types of industry in the economy. Starting out
with a title that denoted an interest in the medicine of rural economy,
it assumed others which introduced the terms "economist" and "industrial
economy" on its masthead.[57] Almost from the very beginning, it promised
studies of occupational disease, including, in some cases, descriptions
of hospital treatment:

> *Le Médecin du peuple*, desiring to be of use to all
> classes of society, has had necessarily to turn
> its attention to the working class, in order to
> indicate the diseases produced by the various kinds
> of occupations; but this work was difficult, to
> render it complete it was necessary to visit the
> factories, the workshops, the humble hovel of the
> worker who works at home, to frequent very unhealthful
> places, to gain a better knowledge of everything
> that is pertinent to the subject which we were
> wishing to treat. By visiting the hospitals of the
> capital, we have studied the different diseases of
> the workers who report there every day; we have not
> neglected to make frequent visits to the workshops,
> either in Paris, or in its environs, to ascertain
> with certainty, which occupations force the various
> parts of the body into distorted postures; those that
> require a great development of the body's muscular
> forces, and the diseases that they most generally
> cause.
>   We will especially be concerned with occupations
> in which noxious materials are used, all the occupa-
> tions that are performed in low and humid locations,
> and the innumerable diseases that these deadly places
> cause artisans who are obliged to spend part of their
> existence in them. We will try to indicate to them
> protective [measures]; and to add some variety to our
> subject, we will enter into some detail on the methods
> by which these occupations are practiced, [since] so-
> ciety people are generally ignorant of how the things
> that they use every day are made.[58]

The concern was, of course, older. Ramazzini's classic study, however, had not been immediately followed by detailed examinations of workers' diseases, but in France, at least, as the eighteenth century progressed, the plates in the *Encyclopédie*, showing people at work without giving any notion of its realities (the workers, like their tools, are depicted quite anonymously and interchangeably) were succeeded by studies and references that expanded Diderot's direct allusions to the vicious effects of most kinds of work on workers' bodies.[59] By the time the 1820s series on occupational diseases appeared, a distinctive way of approaching them was already in evidence. For a time, many physicians tended to assume that work would permanently divide mankind into two unequal classes and that there was little workers could do, apart from voluntarily giving up work that was injurious to them. There seems to be some evidence as well that, in some cases, physicians were prepared to dispute the right of manufacturers and other employers to endanger the atmosphere by releasing noxious substances.

At this stage in my research, it is too early to say if the concerns of *Le Médecin du peuple* formed a uniform continuum of comment linking the earlier works on occupational disease[60] and the later ones which would appear with mounting frequency in the *Annales d'hygiène publique et de médécine légale*, the first number of which appeared in 1829. A brief look at the period covered by the life of the *Médécin du peuple* reveals what occupations attracted the attention of the physicians. They included workers manufacturing white lead and lead salts; laundresses bringing home their laundry to be dried in their own rooms; bakers; porters or janitors; butchers; glassmakers; masons, stone cutters, and plasterers; printers; dockworkers and workers carrying heavy loads.[61] We are still, it seems, in a pre-industrial world. To the workers whose occupations were burdening their lives with chronic disease precious little advice was given, chiefly the need to take precautions at work. For example, bakers were told to cover their mouths with handkerchiefs to reduce the inhalation of flour dust. Because of their work, they usually ended their days in hospitals suffering from pleurisy, peri-pneumonia, and chronic and acute catarrh, aggravated by alcohol. The advice was almost invariably condescendingly didactic, with a lot of stress on personal cleanliness, improved diet, and bursts of alarm that workers were neglecting their health. From time to time, the owners of workshops were admonished, as in the case of printing establishments, to locate their presses above ground level to improve ventilation, and to provide seats for compositors.[62]

But the physician-writers in the same journal were unabasedly committed to industrial change governed by some of Smith's economic principles and the morality of utilitarianism. Surveys of work hazards and
the chronic occupational diseases of a largely non-mechanized economy
were published alongside articles lavishing praise on the wonders of
steam-powered machines, the civilizing effects of the division of la-
bour, and the global expansion of trade. To their chagrin, these developments were not transforming France quickly enough.[63] Material advances were inevitable and, as it was daily becoming clearer, were dependent on a proper understanding of the "laws which preside over the
movement of society." These were not de Gérando's laws, which, as we
saw, were not exclusively economic. By contrast, the writer of this
piece confidently boasted that "Economic knowledge can reveal the real
relations linking men in society." Social prosperity would be ensured
when men came to know the correct connections between the individual
and the general interest: the merchant, the manufacturer, the capitalist, and the landed proprietor, by calculating their risks and their
gains, were working towards the progress of mankind.[64] What they were
achieving was being matched by the progress of medical theory and practice in the thirty or so years since the turn of the century, the proof
of which was discernible, they claimed, in the rise of Europe's population[65] and the "immense" improvements in hospital care and treatment,
due mainly to the applications of chemistry, as well as most of the
other reforms that had been part of the hospital debate for the preceding two generations.[66] With mendicity severely controlled through the
use of *dépôts de mendicité*, which were urged to take as their model a
Bordeaux workshop supported by private funds, "utility, justice, and
truth for all"[67] would at last become the reigning principles of society. One scholar, thinking of the absence of a real change in therapeutic effectiveness, has called much of the medical talk a kind of
"bluff."[68] Vaccination, which did make a lot of headway, and was therefore an exception was, however, not a hospital activity.

Yet the thought of most medical men in France was accurately captured in this optimistic prediction. They believed they were in the
process of strengthening their claims to be the authoritative agents of
normalization in the medical and other domains of life. The hesitations
of the earlier generations of doctors had been dissipated, or at least
their successors revealed fewer of them. We must, in addition, note
that however much they had strengthened their grasp over the processes

of normalization and its disciplinary instruments, the grip remained
paradoxically tenuous and light. For example, where authority lay in
the hospital--with the physicians, the administration, or the nursing
sisters--was a problem expressed with greater frequency during the Revolution and which continued for decades thereafter. The true nature of
clinical instruction raised the extent of medical authority in another
way; for example, what were its practical links with the rate of cure?
The complaint in 1817 by Dr. Nacquart, a member of the Commission of the
Société de Médecine in Paris, who had been offering free consultations
since 1797, that science was not being served for lack of a sufficient
number of observations, is not unconnected with the purpose of clinical
observation, and was certainly not unique.[69] Workers, for the most
part, were admitted to hospitals in the largest centres with perhaps no
greater expectation of cure and recovery than a generation earlier,[70]
but even when cures were achieved, workers returned, if lucky, to work
that was as wasting as before. *La Lancette française*, which kept an eye
on hospital statistics and clinical medicine, claimed in 1830, without
making any connection between them, that mortality rates had declined,
but that the pressure on the Paris Hôtel-Dieu from sick and indigent
workers had been lessened by firm action on the part of the prefect of
the Seine who was sending jobless workers back to their homes in the
provinces.[71] The division between hospital and home care was never
satisfactorily resolved. Medical care was in fact increasingly subject
to chronic breakdown in an economy suffering from recurrent bouts of
collapse. Moreover, if my examination of medical strategies concerning
occupational disease is a measure of their true nature, it was also apparent that doctors could do very little to deal with them.

     The difficulties in making connections between preventive and re-
medial medicine were enormous. To stress the first meant looking more
closely at the social and economic structures underlying disease patterns, with their distinctive power relationships, and consequently
opening up the possibility of widening the bases for a critique of them.
Once occupational and other chronic disease was seen, not only as a
"biological statement about the poor," but as a "social statement,"[72]
the questions of public and private hygiene to which many doctors turned
their attention forced them to raise questions of priority. What should
constitute the mandate and reach of public health? Should emphasis be
put on housing and sanitation, or should the introduction of technological innovations together with public health measures in the work place

be given first call on public funds? As we have seen, the idea of going
into homes to instruct and to use various means of persuasion which did
not stop short of humiliation and ridicule, was considered more practical and fruitful than cumulative intervention in shops, mines, construction sites, and factories. This is not to say that the latter were
totally neglected. That was obviously not the case, but if the ravages
of certain kinds of work could not be ignored, then ways in which medical men, public officials, and publicists investigated the direct and
indirect consequences of work, and the conclusions they were prepared to
draw from their explorations, require closer scrutiny.

What we may say is that men and women were thinking of their illnesses as the tribute they were paying for the privilege of working.
The precise mental processes which gave their betters their understanding of occupational disease, diagnosing them as a "natural" or as a
social process, assigning specificity, taking predisposing factors into
account, and so on, must again await further study. The workers, on the
other hand, carried the visible marks of their infirmities with them,
and if they could do nothing to prevent or to extinguish them, they
could express their sense of themselves in other ways. The year 1830
and the years following constituted a period of revolutionary and quasi-
revolutionary protest in many parts of France. It is not surprising
that the protest strengthened, rather than lessened, the convictions of
doctors and their allies that their social construction of reality and
the strategies they were devising to express them were not only correct,
but needed even firmer support.

Fear of the explosive world of workers was derived from a perspective of work which failed to discern the less visible sources of working-class self-esteem. The various manifestations of working-class
satisfaction, including companionship and mutual respect, were more than
likely rooted in self-worth developed in work that commanded respect.
The numbing effects of many kinds of work were, however, more ubiqui-
tous, overpowering the positive features of the relationship of the
worker to his work and to his fellow-workers. What was exposed to view
were mainly the socially irresponsible or politically riotous expressions of working-class mutuality. That much work had few if any re-
deeming qualities was no secret. But work as a natural function and a
social necessity was advanced as an argument to mitigate its less desirable consequences. Attentive readers of Adam Smith knew that the division of labor was not a stimulus to the mind; only that it increased

productivity. Utilizing the more optimistic of Smith's arguments, some observers, as we saw, capitulated eagerly to the promises of technology. Others were far less certain, but wavered between schemes of self-help and franker appeals for discipline, because they had difficulty in expressing belief in working-class capacity to achieve enduring independence based on family affection and loyalty. Indeed, they did not find it easy to locate the sources of affect in the working-class family, and they found it even harder to locate its reservoirs of discipline. They nevertheless conceded that such qualities might exist under the manifest primitive, self-destructive, and socially destructive feelings of the working-class, or perhaps they more easily assumed that such qualities could, at least partially, be imposed upon it. In more confident mood, they recalled that work had always been socially divisive. The various compensatory devices of a paternalistic and deferential society had obscured the fullest consequences of social tension, and at the same time encouraged belief in the emotional impoverishment of workers. As work became more debilitating in many unprecedented ways during this transitional period, the idea of preserving the working-class family according to a pre-industrial model was replaced by an attempt to construct a working-class version of a middle-class abstraction. But if the aim was the improvement of the working-class family's condition, it stopped short of any change that would alter the position of the social classes.

Foucault is confident that the authorities alone constructed the context in which shifts in attitude occurred or change was managed. He tends to overestimate the clarity of their intentions and the firmness of their purpose. As we have seen, the gaps between their theoretical and practical grasp of the problems they tried to face were often quite staggering. Conversely, he underestimates the power of the "manipulable" groups to challenge the premises of the authorities by concealing the opaque sources of their skills, not only to survive but to have some understanding of their own bodies and minds caught in the toils of work.

NOTES

1 Three of Foucault's works are especially pertinent for the present
   study. I list only the translated versions: *The Birth of the Clin-
   ic: An Archaeology of Medical Perception*, trans. A. M. Sheridan
   Smith. (New York, 1973); *Discipline and Punish. The Birth of the
   Prison*, trans. A. Sheridan (New York, 1977); *The History of Sexuality
   I: An Introduction*, trans. R. Hurley (New York, 1978).

2 For a critique of Ivan Illich's thesis that the medical profession
   determines the nature of medical and related forms of control and
   authority independently of other socially dominant groups, see V.
   Navarro, "The Industrialization of Fetishism or the Fetishism of
   Industrialization. A Critique of Ivan Illich," *Social Science and
   Medicine*, 9 (1975), 351-63.

3 See Charles Taylor's first chapter in his *Hegel* (Cambridge, 1975) on
   the idea of progress. Hannah Arendt provides a keen and perceptive
   glimpse of the kind of demonic force that has permeated the work of
   scientists in the study published after her death, *The Life of the
   Mind* (2 vols., New York, 1978), esp. I: *Thinking*, pp. 54-55 and II:
   Knowing, pp. 152-54. The debate over the promise and boundaries of
   science may be sampled in "Limits of Scientific Inquiry," *Daedalus*,
   107 (Spring, 1978). Gunther S. Stent, *Paradoxes of Progress* (San
   Francisco, 1978) also questions the unlimited belief in scientific
   progress and uses the critical term "scientism." So does Joseph Ben-
   David, *The Scientist's Role in Society. A Comparative Study* (Englewood Cliffs, 1971), who discusses its eighteenth-century roots. For
   a valuable discussion of "scientism" as it has figured in the work of
   social and political theorists in Europe and in the U.S., see R. J.
   Bernstein, *The Restructuring of Social and Political Theory* (New
   York, 1976).

4 In an unpublished paper "Medicine and the Enlightenment in Eighteenth-
   Century England," presented to the Society for the Social History of
   Medicine (U.K.), Hull, July 1979, Roy Porter criticized historians
   who would, in his words, hypostatize such cultural values as health
   and disease, but he does not consider the extent to which theorists
   and practitioners in the eighteenth century and in the next also did
   so.

5 Among the vast literature on public relief and the French hospitalization movement, see the work of George Rosen, some of whose essays
   have been collected in *From Medical Police to Social Medicine*; *Essays
   on the History of Health Care* (New York, 1974); *Madness in Society.
   Chapters in the Historical Sociology of Mental Illness* (New York,
   1968); and Louis Greenbaum's exceedingly valuable articles on the
   French old régime hospitals: "The Commercial Treaty of Humanity. La
   tournée des hôpitaux anglais par Jacques Tenon en 1789," *Revue
   d'histoire des sciences*, 24, (1971), 317-50; "Jean-Sylvain Bailly,
   the baron de Breteuil and 'Four New Hospitals of Paris,'" *Clio
   Medica*, 8 (1973), 261-84; "Tempest in the Academy. Jean-Baptiste Le
   Roy, the Paris Academy of Sciences and the Project of a New Hôtel-
   Dieu," *Archives internationales d'Histoire des Sciences*, 24 (1974),
   122-40; "'Measure of Civilization': The Hospital Thought of Jacques

Tenon on the Eve of the French Revolution," *Bulletin of the History
of Medicine*, 49 (1975), 43-56; "Health-Care and Hospital-Building in
Eighteenth-Century France: Reform Proposals of du Pont de Nemours
and Condorcet," *Studies on Voltaire and the Eighteenth Century* (hereafter *SVEC* 153 (1976), 895-930.

6 "Plan pour la suppression de l'hôtel-Dieu et l'établissement de neuf
   hospices, présenté par le sieur Nicolson, avocat, 17 mai 1790," in
   A. Tuetey ed., *L'assistance publique à Paris pendant la Révolution*
   (4 vols., 1895-97), I, 113.

7 "Rapport sur l'organisation générale des secours publics," 12 vendémiaire an IV (October 4, 1795), in *ibid.*, III, 127.

8 Jacques Tenon, *Mémoires sur les hôpitaux de Paris* (Paris, 1788).
   Firm and reliable figures for the number of hospitals of all kinds
   in France before the Revolution do not exist. The *Comité de mendicité* in 1790 claimed that there were 2,185 *hôpitaux généraux*, which
   were establishments taking in most marginal and deviant groups, the
   figure used by Tenon himself. See "Opinion de M. Tenon...sur la
   réunion des deux comités de mendicité et de salubrité," Assembleé
   nationale, October 14, 1791. Olwen H. Hufton, *The Poor of
   Eighteenth-Century France 1750-1789* (Oxford, 1974), p. 143, 143n,
   thinks the figure is exaggerated, and contrasts it with the Comité's
   own confirmed figures totalling 1,438 *hôpitaux* and hôtels-Dieu. For
   the most trustworthy recent attempt to sort out the different classes
   of hospital establishment, see M. Jeorger, "La structure hospitalière
   de la France sous l'ancien régime," *Annales E.S.C.*, 32 (Sept.-Oct.,
   1977), 1025-51.

9 For the history of the Academy's recommendations to build the four
   hospitals, see Greenbaum's articles, cited above. The recommendations did not come to fruition, because the government in 1788, just
   before the political crisis became intense, earmarked the funds for
   hospital construction for other purposes. The present author has
   looked at how the hospital question during this period was part of
   the movement towards the technologization and depoliticization of
   French society, in "Politics in the Service of Knowledge: The Debate
   over the Administration of Welfare and Medicine in Late Eighteenth-
   Century France" *Social History* forthcoming. See also his review
   article, "Politics, Power and Psychiatry: A Review of *L'ordre psychiatrique: L'âge d'or de l'aliénisme* by Robert Castel," *International Journal of Law and Psychiatry*, II (1979), 249-61.

10 C. Bloch, *L'assistance et l'état en France à la veille de la Révolution* (Paris, 1908).

11 For a sampling see the archives of the *Sociéte Royale de Médecine*
   (hereafter SRM), Académie Nationale de Médecine, Paris. Bloch,
   L'assistance, has collected materials from various *cahiers*, a major
   source. SRM 130-133 includes a number of memoirs ranging in date
   from 1771 to 1791, from correspondents in cities like Grenoble,
   Paris, and Dijon, and smaller places such as St. Etienne-en-Forez,
   Séguenville, Morlaix, and Pontoise.

12 The phrase is used by E. M. Sigsworth, "Gateway to Death? Medicine,
   Hospitals and Mortality, 1700-1850," in P. Mathias, ed., *Science and
   Society, 1600-1900* (Cambridge, 1972).

13   See, for example, my study, "Rationality and Control in French
     Eighteenth-Century Medical Views of the Peasantry," *Comparative
     Studies in Society and History*, 21 (January 1979), 82-112. For an
     attempt to calculate the number of practitioners in the decade be-
     fore the Revolution, see J. P. Goubert, "The Extent of Medical Prac-
     tice in France around 1780," *Journal of Social History* 10 (1976-77),
     410-27.

14   See D. B. Weiner, "Le droit de l'homme à la santé--Une belle ideé
     devant l'assemblée constituante: 1790-1791," *Clio Medica*, 5 (1970),
     209-23.

15   Tenon, *Mémoires*, p. 278.

16   François Doublet, "Hospice de Charité, année 1788," *Journal de méde-
     cine, chirurgie, pharmacie*, 82 (1790), 193-234. Doublet also col-
     lected the *Observations faites dans le département des hôpitaux
     civils* (4 vols., Paris, 1785-1788), which originally appeared in the
     above-cited journal. For another valuable study of hospital mortal-
     ity figures, see SRM 134, Dr. W. Munniks, "Des moyens pour détruire
     des abus qui s'opposent à la conservation des enfans en France, et
     qui pourront en même temps contribuer à fortifier les tempéramens
     des générations présentes et futures, August 31, 1784."

17   I completed the present study before I could benefit fully from K.
     Figlio's article, "Sinister Medicine? A Critique of Left Approaches
     to Medicine," *Radical Science Journal*, no. 9 (1979), 14-68, 148-60.
     His remarks, 29-31, 50-51, on the hospitals are similar to my own.

18   See my article, "Rationality and Control," for references to the
     literature on these subjects. Two studies which should not be over-
     looked are those by T. Gelfand, "Medical Practitioners and Charla-
     tans. The Comité de Salubrité Enquête of 1790-91," *Histoire
     Sociale-Social History*, 11 (1978), 62-97; and C. C. Hannaway,
     "Veterinary Medicine and Rural Health Care in Pre-Revolutionary
     France," *Bulletin of the History of Medicine*, 51 (1977), 431-47.

19   What can only be described as testaments of faith in their power to
     benefit mankind may be seen in the following: F. Vicq d'Azyr,
     Oeuvres, ed. by J. L. Moreau de la Sarthe (6 vols., Paris, 1805), V,
     64; SRM 115, Pierre Flandrin, "Mémoire sur cette question: Quelle
     est la meilleure manière d'enseigner la médecine clinique dans un
     hôpital?" Lent 1793; P. -J. -G. Cabanis, *Coup d'oeil sur les révolu-
     tions et sur la réforme de la médecine*, in C. Lehec and J. Caze-
     neuve, eds., *Oeuvres philosophiques de Cabanis* (2 vols., Paris,
     1956) (hereafter OP); the contributors to Fourcroy's shortlived
     journal, *La médecine éclairée par les sciences physiques* (1791-92).
     See also Daniel Roche, "Talents, Raison et sacrifice: l'image du
     médecin des Lumières d'après les éloges de la Société Royale de
     Médecine (1776-1789)," *Annales E.S.C.*, 32 (1977), 866-86 and his *Le
     siècle des lumières en province. Académies et académiciens provin-
     ciaux 1680-1789* (2 vols., Paris, The Hague, 1978), I, 243-45, 372-
     75.

20   To cite a later example of the importance attributed to clinical in-
     struction in hospital ideology, Dr. Alphonse Leroy, professor in the
     Faculty of Medicine in Paris, urged in 1791 the establishment of a
     school devoted to the theory and practice of obstetrics, gynecology,

and children's illnesses. See "Rapport au Conseil municipal sur le plan d'une Ecole de Médecine et d'Accouchements présenté par M. Alphonse Leroy," Feb. 12, 1791, in Tuetey, *L'assistance publique*, I, 59-63.

21 Foucault, *Birth of the Clinic*, p. 42.

22 Nicholas Chambon de Montaux, *Moyens de rendre les hôpitaux plus utiles à la nation* (Paris, 1787). Cf. "Copie du projet d'enseignment de médecine pratique par M. Chambon," October 23, 1789 in SRM 115. T. Gelfand has published an assessment of Chambon, "A Clinical Ideal: Paris 1789," *Bulletin of the History of Medicine*, 51 (1977), 397-411.

23 See C. Bloch and A. Tuetey, *Procès-verbaux et rapports du Comité de mendicité de la Constituante (1790-1791)* (Paris, 1911), pp. 393-96. If a comparison is made between the Comité's fourth report and the section in Cabanis's II, esp. 44-45, devoted to home care, the wording is found to be often identical. Cabanis was a member of the Paris Committee on Hospitals from 1791 to 1792. He was closely connected with M. -A. Thouret, who was a member of the *Comité* and who was to become director of the Faculty of Medicine when it was set up again in 1794 under the name of Ecole de Santé. M. S. Staum's excellent study, *Cabanis. Enlightenment and Medical Philosophy in the French Revolution* (Princeton, 1980), which appeared too late for me to consult thoroughly, treats Cabanis's thought on the hospital question on pp. 136-146.

24 Chambon, *Moyens*. Cf. Foucault, *The Birth of the Clinic*, p. 85, who calls this a régime of "economic freedom."

25 Du Pont de Nemours, *Idées sur les secours à donner aux pauvres malades dans une grande ville* (Philadelphia, 1786). See Greenbaum, *SVEC*, for a fuller discussion of Dupont's views.

26 L. -S. Mercier, *Tableau de Paris* (8 vols., Amsterdam, 1782-83), I, 150-161, 235-28; II, 197-98.

27 See J. Lecuir, "Criminalité et 'moralité': Montyon, statisticien du Parlement de Paris," *Revue d'histoire moderne et contemporaine*, 21 (July-Sept. 1974), 445-93. What impressed Richard Cobb in his study of the poor who ended up in the morgue as suicides or as accident victims in the 1790s is that they belonged to a "very static form of society, its immutability reinforced and perpetuated by family relationships, marriage, common provincial or Parisian origins...and hereditary occupations," *Death in Paris* (Oxford, 1978), p. 13. Cobb is referring to people whose occupations were "essential to the continuation of everyday life...," such as carters, porters, stable-boys, water-carriers, chimney sweeps, laundresses, and so on, but not domestic servants. These people were, it would seem, as much concerned to maintain family and kinship ties as the artisans.

28 For a valuable discussion of the notion of the domicile in French law, see A. -J. Arnaud, *Essai d'analyse structurale du code civil français. La règle du jeu dans la paix bourgeoise* (Paris, 1973), pp. 60-61, 72, 84.

29 On Cabanis's position, see Staum, *Cabanis*, pp. 140-44. A good ex-
    ample of how the poor were compelled to meet residence qualifica-
    tions is to be found in Delecloy's recommendations on public assis-
    tance in Paris. See Tuetey, *L'assistance publique*, III, 128, Arti-
    cle 6, which deals with Paris. The strong stress and reliance on
    local attestations of worthiness, the rôle of the parish priest in
    determining it, and the specific responsibilities of local notables
    in the distribution of assistance, were constant themes during the
    old régime. There were many proposals in which certification by the
    curé for relief eligibility is set side by side with the expanded
    rôle which physicians wanted for themselves. For examples, see
    Archives nationales (hereafter AN), F[16]936. The *curé's* claims dur-
    ing the aftermath of the Civil Constitution of the Clergy were for-
    feited, but the authority of local notables survived. In 1789, the
    "Dames de Miséricorde" in Paris, the wives of men in commerce, bank-
    ing, finance, and the professions, were called upon to help the in-
    digent. See Archives de l'Assistance Publique (hereafter AAP),
    A-1205[2], M. -J. -J. Menuret de Chambaud, *Essai sur les secours à
    donner aux malades pauvres. Par le moyen de petits hôpitaux multi-
    pliés* (Paris, 1789), pp. 33-43. During the Convention, the wives of
    the commissioners of relief in a Paris section were also asked to
    care for the poor sick. See M. Chiron, "Au Comité de l'Indivisi-
    bilité en 1793. La Bienfaisance sous la Commune révolutionnaire,"
    in *Bulletin de la Société amicale d'études des Bureaux de bien-
    faisance de Paris*, no. 2 (1904), 36-47. An *officier de santé* at
    Bordeaux demanded that all women be forced to overcome their aver-
    sion for the poor. See AN, F[17]1359, dossier 3, pièce 169, J. -F.
    Capelle, *Des temples de l'humanité ou les hospices régenérés* (Bor-
    deaux, no date). On continuity of control by notables during the
    Revolution, see R. Dreyfus, "Les secours à domicile à Paris pendant
    la Révolution," *La Révolution française*, 48 (1905), 490-511, esp.
    504. His article provides some information on the mechanics of
    distribution, as does the study by M. Fosseyeux, "Les Comités de
    bienfaisance des sections du Finistère et du Panthéon," *ibid.*, 60
    (1911), 504-35.

30 *Premier rapport fait au nom du Comité de salut public. Sur les
    moyens d'extirper la mendicité dans les campagnes, et sur les se-
    cours que doit accorder la République aux citoyens indigens*, Con-
    vention nationale, 22 floréal an II (May 11, 1794). At the very
    time that Barère was citing his poverty statistics, a count of the
    number of people eligible for relief in the Finistère section in
    Paris showed that over half of its population of nearly 11,000
    needed help. See Fosseyeux, "Les comités," 520-21, 529.

31 His views are to be found in AN, F[16]936 in a memorandum to the
    Comité de mendicité.

32 J. B. Delecloy, *Rapport sur l'organisation des secours publics*,
    Convention nationale, 12 vendémiaire an IV (October 4, 1795).

33 Delaporte, *Rapport au nom de la commission de l'organisation des
    secours publics, Conseil des Cinq-Cents*, 13 messidor an IV (July 1,
    1796).

34 *Ibid.*

35 Delaporte, *Rapport au nom de la commission des hospices. Secours aux hospices civils et aux enfans de la patrie, Conseil des Cinq-Cents*, 24 thermidor an VI (Aug. 10, 1798).

36 *Extrait du registre des délibérations du Directoire exécutif. Le Directoire exécutif au Conseil des Cinq-Cents, Conseil des Cinq-Cents*, 26 nivôse an VI (January 15, 1798).

37 *Rapport présenté au Directoire exécutif par le ministre de l'Intérieur*, 26 nivôse an VI (January 15, 1798).

38 Jouenne, *Rapport fait au nom d'une commission spéciale, sur les messages du Directoire exécutif, relatifs aux hospices civils, Conseil des Cinq-Cents*, 9 ventôse an VII (February 27, 1799).

39 Delecloy, *Rapport fait au nom d'une commission spéciale, sur la résolution du 22 germinal an VII, relative à l'administration des hospices civils, Conseil des Anciens, 9 messidor au VIII* (June 27, 1799); Porcher, *Opinion de Porcher, sur la résolution du 26 germinal an VII, relative aux hospices, Conseil des Anciens*, 16 messidor an VII, (July 4, 1799).

40 Delecloy, *ibid.*

41 See, for example, *Réflexions sur les hôpitaux et particulièrement sur ceux de la Commune de Paris et l'établissement du Mont-de-Piété*, par un employé du ministère de l'Intérieur (Paris, an VIII), *Rapports au Conseil-général des hospices, sur les hôpitaux et hospices, le secours à domicile...*par MM. Camus et Duquesnoy (Paris, an XI).

42 See Castel, *L'ordre psychiatrique*, pp. 76-84 for another reading of this problem.

43 *Projet d'établissement d'une Société bienfaisante des orphelins abandonnés, adressé au Département des établissements publics* par M. André-Jean de la Rocque, premier commis à la Mairie, in Tuetey, *L'assistance publique*, I, 51-57. De la Rocque's two projects were *Avantages des caisses établies en faveur des veuves dans plusieurs gouvernements* (Paris, 1787) and *Etablissement d'une caisse générale des épargnes du peuple, susceptible d'exécution dans les principaux gouvernements de l'Europe* (Brussels or Paris, 1785 or 1787).

44 S. Kaplan, "Réflexions sur la police du monde du travail, 1700-1815," *Revue historique*, 256 (1979), 17-78, calls the repression of working-class activities, although dressed up in the name of individual liberty, a transparent vestige of the older fears.

45 AN, F^{15}3963, Société philanthropique. Du procès-verbal de la séance du comité d'administration de la Société philanthropique, du 12 thermidor an XII (July 31, 1803).

46 Reports by Dupont, *Rapports et comptes rendus de la Société philanthropique de Paris, pendant l'an XII*, p. 99. Cited in M. Sibalis, "Workers' Organizations in Napoleonic Paris," *Proceedings of the Fifth Annual Meeting of the Western Society for French History* edited by J. D. Falk (Santa Barbara, 1978), p. 221. Cf. J. J. McLain, *The Economic Writings of Du Pont de Nemours* (Newark and London, 1977), pp. 128-41, 164-65, 183-85, 192.

47   AN, F^{15}2738, Rapport à Sa Majesté l'Empereur Roi sur les sociétés
     de prévoyance, no date.

48   *Ibid.*

49   Archives de l'Assistance Publique, A-2167^{16}, *Association de bien-
     faisance mutuelle formée en janvier 1809* (Paris, 1819).

50   AN, F^{15}3963, *Rapport annuel fait le 31 janvier 1810, à l'assemblée
     générale de la Société d'assistance charitable.*

51   See J. -M. de Gérando, *Le Visiteur du pauvre* (Paris, 1820). For a
     discussion of his thought in the Idéologue tradition, see S. Mor-
     avia, *Il pensiero degli idéologues. Scienza e filosofia in Francia
     (1780-1815)* (Florence, 1974), esp. pp. 415-56. On the family as an
     entity requiring discipline and moral instruction, see I. Joseph,
     P. Fritsch, and A. Battegay, *Disciplines à domicile. L'édification
     de la famille. Recherches*, no. 28 (Fontenay-sous-Bois, 1977). Cf. J.
     Donzelot, *La police des familles* (Paris, 1977). For a critique of
     Donzelot, see M. Mérignas, "Travail social et structures de classe.
     A propos de 'La police des familles' de J. Donzelot," in *Critiques
     de l'économie politique*, no. 3 (April-June 1978), 24-56.

52   See for examples of their concerns and influence, K. A. Lynch, "The
     Problem of Child Labor Reform and the Working-Class Family in France
     during the July Monarchy," *Proceedings of the Fifth Annual Meeting
     of the Western Society for French History*, edited by J. D. Falk
     (Santa Barbara, 1978), 228-36. In the same volume, see A. F. La
     Berge, "A Restoration Prefect and Public Health: Alban de Ville-
     neuve-Bargemont at Nantes and Lille, 1824-30," 128-37. See also A.
     F. La Berge, "The Paris Health Council, 1802-1848," *Bulletin of the
     History of Medicine*, 49 (1975), 339-52; D. B. Weiner, "Public Health
     under Napoleon: the Conseil de Salubrité de Paris, 1802-1815,"
     Clio Medica, 9 (1974), 271-84; A. Berman, "J.B.A. Chevallier,
     Pharmacist-Chemist: A Major Figure in Nineteenth-Century French
     Public Health," *Bulletin of the History of Medicine*, 52 (1978),
     200-213.

53   A. Cuvillier, ed., *Un journal d'ouvriers: "L'Atelier" (1840-1850)*
     (Paris, 1954), p. 44.

54   T. Adorno, "Sociology and Psychology," *New Left Review*, 46 (Nov.-
     Dec. 1967), 71.

55   For a full and excellent discussion of the cluster of ideas on the
     environment, see L. J. Jordanova, "Earth Science and Environmental
     Evidence: The Synthesis of the Late Enlightenment," *British Society
     for the History of Science Monographs*, I (1979), 119-46.

56   See A. F. La Berge, "The Physician-Hygienists of Lyon and Public
     Health, 1815-1848," an unpublished paper delivered at the 1979 meet-
     ing of the Society for French Historical Studies.

57   Its successive names were *Hygie, Journal de médecine, d'économie
     domestique et rurale; Nouvelle hygie, journal de médecine, d'écono-
     mie domestique et rurale; Le Médecin du peuple, journal de santé et
     d'économie domestique et rurale; and L'Economiste ou le Médecin du
     peuple, Journal de santé, d'économie publique, industrielle, domes-
     tique et rurale.*

58 *Le Médecin du peuple*, March 9, 1828.

59 See the excellent articles by J. Proust, "L'image du peuple au
    travail dans les planches de l'Encyclopédie," in *Images du peuple
    au dix-huitième siècle* (Paris, 1973), 65-85; G. Besse, "Aspects du
    travail ouvrier au XVIIIe siècle en France," in J. Pappas, ed.,
    Essays on Diderot and the Enlightenment in Honor of Otis Fellows
    (Geneva, 1974), 71-88.

60 A. Farge, "Les artisans malades de leur travail," *Annales E.S.C.*,
    32 (1977), 993-1006, offers a brief look at the prevailing atti-
    tudes towards occupational disease at the end of the eighteenth
    century. There is much work to be done in this aspects of social
    medicine, and I am pursuing research in it. Two studies touch on
    occupational disease incidentally. The first is A. E. Imhof, "The
    Hospital in the 18th Century: For Whom?" *Journal of Social His-
    tory*, 10 (1976-77), 448-70. The second is by C. Webster, "The Crisis
    of the Hospitals during the Industrial Revolution," *International
    Congress of the History of Science, Actes 15e 1977* (1978), 214-23.

61 Respectively appearing in *Hygie*, Dec. 2., 1825; *Le Médecin du
    peuple*, March 16, April 13, May 4, 1828; *L'Economiste*, June 1, June
    15, July 20, Aug. 31, Nov. 2, 1828.

62 For references, see *Le Médecin du peuple*, April 13, 1828; *L'Econo-
    miste*, May 25, July 20, Aug. 24, Aug. 31, Nov. 30, 1828.

63 *Ibid.*, May 18, June 29, Sept. 7, 21, 1828.

64 *Ibid.*, Jan. 4, 1829.

65 *Nouvelle hygie*, Nov. 18, 1827.

66 *L'Economiste*, July 6, 1828.

67 *Ibid.*, Sept. 21, 28, 1828.

68 J. Léonard, "L'historien et le philosophe. A propos de 'Surveiller
    et punir. Naissance de la prison,'" *Annales historiques de la
    Révolution française*, 49 (1977), 163-81. Compare what R. C. Fox
    has termed the modern "'mystique,' cultivated by physicians them-
    selves through their claim that they command knowledge and skills
    that are too esoteric to be freely and fully shared with lay per-
    sons," in "The Medicalization and Demedicalization of American So-
    ciety," *Daedalus*, 106 (Winter 1977), 9-22, esp. 12.

69 A good example of the hostility shown physicians in the hospital may
    be seen in the complaint that they were subjecting patients to
    "experiment for young doctors," so that "an office of consolation
    and cure will be transformed into a ministry of pain and death."
    See "Instructions données par la Direction de l'hospice de charité
    de malades de Toulouse . . . prise au sujet d'une pétition pré-
    sentée par le citoyen Dupau, officier de santé," Feb. 6, 1794, in J.
    Adher, ed., *Recueil de documents sur l'assistance publique dans le
    district de Toulouse de 1789 à 1800*, (Toulouse, 1918), pp. 75-79.
    See L. Greenbaum, "Nurses and Doctors in Conflict: Piety and Medi-
    cine in the Paris Hôtel-Dieu on the Eve of the French Revolution,"
    Clio Medica, 13 (1979), 247-76, for a discussion of the conflicting

aims, but similar power-seeking goals, of physicians and nursing
sisters. Nacquart's report may be seen in *Journal général de
Médecine*, 43 (1812), 13-15. For an examination of the nature of
clinical teaching, see M. Wiriot, *L'enseignement clinique dans les
hôpitaux de Paris entre 1794 et 1848* (Paris, 1970). See the older
study by E. H. Ackerknecht, *Medicine at the Paris Hospital 1794-
1848* (Baltimore, 1967).

70   G. Pons, *Essai de sociologie des malades dans les hôpitaux de Paris
     pendant les années 1815 à 1848* (Zurich, 1969), is hardly adequate.
     It has been roughly estimated that the number of patients admitted
     to the Paris hospitals increased from about 38,000 in 1807 to
     53,000 twenty years later. See Ackerknecht, *Medicine,* p. 18.

71   See *La Lancette française,* II (1830), 387-89, for the claim that
     the mortality rate at the Hôtel-Dieu had fallen from one in three to
     one in six or even seven between 1780 and 1830. Tenon's statistics,
     it will be recalled, gave a mortality figure of one in four and one-
     half. Cf. W. F. Bynum, "Hospital, Disease and Community: The Lon-
     don Fever Hospital, 1801-1850," in C. E. Rosenberg, ed., *Healing and
     History. Essays for George Rosen* (New York, 1979), 97-115, esp.
     108, for his conclusions on the minor if negligible reduction in
     hospital mortality statistics. Mortality, he adds, was *higher* (my
     emphasis) outside the hospital. Nevertheless, he is convinced (111)
     that the "hospital's therapeutic and prophylactic program remained
     fixed for half a century and more."

72   The terms are used by R. Jacoby, *Social Amnesia. A Critique of
     Contemporary Psychology from Adler to Laing* (Boston, 1975), p. 140,
     in his discussion of poverty and chronic disease.

THE DECLINE OF THE ORDINARY PRACTITIONER AND THE RISE OF A MODERN MEDICAL PROFESSION

TOBY GELFAND

I

Introduction

The history of medicine as a profession is currently the subject of considerable attention. Recent studies of the profession in nineteenth-century France and mid-Victorian London by Jacques Léonard and M. Jeanne Peterson respectively have brought new insights and original methodologies to bear on the social structure of medical practitioners.[1] Léonard employs the methods of the Annales school of historiography while Peterson's theoretical approach relies on American sociology of medicine and the professions.[2]

Both illuminate the daily life, work, and career problems of the rank and file of the medical profession in the nineteenth century, an area neglected by medical historians who have dealt largely with the development and achievements of a relatively small medical elite. Thanks to studies such as Léonard's and Peterson's, we are beginning to see a dynamic, full-bodied picture of a profession in the process of emerging as a powerful force in society. We are shown the origins of what will become, according to one's interpretive preference, the "archetypal profession" or the "medical nemesis."[3]

Yet these roots, as Léonard and Peterson vividly demonstrate, were insecurely anchored and frail for most of the nineteenth century. By today's standards, the lot of many, if not most, general medical practitioners was anything but enviable. It was rather a continual struggle to earn a living and to gain a place in respectable society. The actors themselves were often painfully conscious of their ambiguous if not downright marginal economic and social status.

Yet, from a different perspective, that of the structure of the medical professions in Old Régime Europe, the nineteenth-century situation looks novel and modern, if somewhat underdeveloped. I do not mean to say that a starving G.P. in nineteenth-century London was somehow better off than a barber-surgeon in the eighteenth-century French

countryside. In personal terms, misery is irreducibly miserable. This
paper will argue, however, that a sharp historical discontinuity occurred between those I call "ordinary practitioners" and general medical
practitioners.

My major analytic claim is that modern G.P.'s constitute part of a
unified medical profession whereas ordinary practitioners formed an occupational group, separate and distinct from licensed medical doctors.
Although the latter claimed authority over ordinary practitioners, this
claim, for various reasons we will discuss, was largely empty. On the
contrary, ordinary practitioners sometimes competed with medical doctors; in any case medical professional structure before the nineteenth
century was pluralistic, not unified.

Another way of formulating our argument is as follows: modern professional structure is essentially unified, though it was and still is
characterized by stratification resulting in marked socio-economic dis-
parities between the extremes. Nevertheless, the general practitioner
is as modern a figure as the elite specialist against whom he is defined.[4] (The logic of this position and status in a modern medical profession dictated that the G.P. would become in effect a "specialist" in
general practice, a rank officially consecrated in the 1960s by the
adoption of the new title of "family practitioner.") The two poles are
linked by a common fundamental education in terms of knowledge and institutional experience; secondary differences between G.P. and specialist training are differences in degree rather than kind, quantitative
rather than qualitative. Although we tend to notice the differences in
residency training programs as diverse as psychiatry and cardiac surgery, extreme fragmentation is a relatively recent phenomenon and remains subsequent to a shared educational experience. Both G.P. and
specialist stand together on the other side of a gulf from the ordinary
practitioner, a gulf as wide as the economic, social, political, and
cultural transformations separating modern from early modern Europe.

Needless to say, our highly schematized picture of abrupt educational unification distorts historical reality. Ordinary practitioners
did not march blithely toward a holocaust from the ashes of which G.P.'s
and specialists arose. Even in France (which I confess in advance to be
my paradigm case), where the Revolution abolished all existing medical
institutions and simply decreed educational unification, the barber-
surgeons, who were the ordinary practitioners of the Old Régime, survived while a new class of second-level doctors--the officers of
health--came into being.[5]

Although medical professional unification did not eliminate ordinary practitioners suddenly and totally, it did provide a means for their control and systematic reduction in numbers. Nineteenth-century medicine, unlike "new" technical professions such as engineering, developed not primarily by direct expansion but by a process of reducing, purifying, and standardizing its ranks. In France, the Revolution at the end of the eighteenth century marked a decisive turning point. Other countries followed their own distinctive national patterns and the process occurred at different rates and times. Germany eliminated *wundärzte* and feldshers during the course of the nineteenth century; Russia tried to do the same after the Bolshevik Revolution but found she could not do without her feldshers.[6] The British situation was particularly complex and is difficult to pinpoint chronologically. Apothecaries remained an important medical corporation throughout the first half of the nineteenth century, if not beyond. Peterson identifies the period between 1858 and 1886 as crucial for the emergence of a strong, autonomous medical profession. She describes the British profession in 1858 as "a hybrid agglomeration of...physicians, surgeons...and apothecaries" and "not truly a profession."[7] Yet, another social historian of English medicine identifies an earlier period (1830-1858) as "a decisive turning point in medical education in this country" during which "the modern structure of medical education emerged."[8] He concludes in a masterful display of relativistic qualification: "During that period [1830-1858], medical knowledge became more scientific, medical education more systematic, and the medical profession more unified."[9]

Relativism is the snare into which an objective evaluation of medical professional power is likely to fall. Was President Tito's recent last illness illustrative of modern medical power or its weakness? Either alternative could plausibly be defended, depending upon one's basis for comparison. Tito doubtless would not have been able to survive as long as he did without modern heroic measures; yet who would deny that future innovations in therapy will probably make the efforts of his doctors in 1980 look impotent by comparison? The same problem arises with regard to other professional issues besides competence, such as authority over patients or control over the conditions of work in hospitals.

I want to suggest that some of the recent literature drawing attention to the limits of nineteenth-century medical power takes as a

standard for comparison, at least implicitly, some later development, if
not today's situation. When this is done, the nineteenth-century profession inevitably appears relatively poorly trained, disunified, dis-
organized, and weak.

If, instead of looking forward in time for comparisons, we forget
more recent developments (or place them aside insofar as possible) and
look at eighteenth-century professional structure, then another solution
presents itself. We would still have a relativism problem if the
eighteenth-century situation appeared as simply a pallid version of
nineteenth-century medicine. On the other hand, if eighteenth-century
professional structure can be shown to be qualitatively different, then
we have a basis for identifying some of the key variables in the transformation process.

In what follows, I shall first outline an abstract model of ordinary practitioners, then flesh out this model with examples from the
eighteenth-century French medical world and, finally, suggest some reasons for the decline of this type of practitioner and the emergence of a
modern profession.

II

Ordinary Practitioners: a Model

The components of our model of ordinary practitioners include the
following: (1) official legal status as a member of an occupational
group, typically a guild or corporation, such as apothecaries or barber-
surgeons; (2) substantial numerical strength with levels of medical density approaching 1 practitioner per 1,000 inhabitants; this contrasts
sharply with the relatively few practitioners in the upper stratum
(doctors of medicine); (3) wide geographical distribution reaching out
to small rural villages; (4) modest to low social origins, status, and
aspirations comparable to those of skilled artisans; (5) training by apprenticeship, a private contractual arrangement binding the master and
the apprentice's family; subsequent training by further private arrangements as opposed to public settings such as schools and hospitals;
(6) comprehensive practice embracing various aspects of internal medicine, surgery, pharmacy, and other activities related to bodily care but
not considered part of medicine today (barber's work, other grooming and
cosmetic attentions, baths, massage, etc.); (7) constitution of an effectively independent corps of practitioners. Despite nominal

subordination to medical faculties, the ordinary practitioners have
their own group identity and training structures. They thus have a degree of autonomy and a potential for serious intraprofessional competition and conflict; (8) a practitioner-patient relationship with considerable discretionary powers resting with the client or patient. These
typically include not only choice of practitioner and whether to comply
with his advice, but an active role in determining the conditions and
even the content of the medical task. At higher social levels, this
relationship may be described as a patronage system in which a wealthy
patron retains a personal doctor for his health needs just as he might
hire an artist for aesthetic projects. The patron fixes goals and makes
decisions based on his own understanding of the matters at hand and the
technical suggestions of his professional adviser.[10] At the lower end
of the social scale--for instance, a peasant calling a country barber-
surgeon for a phlebotomy--the power relationships are analogous, though
the problem may be greatly simplified from that which prompted the
aristocrat to call his physician. In the final analysis, however, the
practitioner-patient relationship, in both instances, is one in which
the patient's wishes and values shape the transaction. In both instances too, one could say that the patient seeks a practitioner who
will share his viewpoint. Thus, a social fit between practitioner and
patient takes on particular importance; a matching process occurs between extraordinary physicians and extraordinary clients, on the one
hand, and between ordinary practitioners and ordinary patients on the
other.

III

Ordinary Practitioners in Eighteenth-century France: Barber-Surgeons

A. Official Status

Barber-surgeons enjoyed recognized legal status as members of
communautés, professional societies constituted along the lines of
guilds and possessing statutory codes.[11] Each *communauté* had the right
to confer degrees to prospective surgeons within a specific geographical
region. The *communauté* conducted examinations according to its statutes
and was responsible for the regulation [*police*] of practice in the region. The statutes defined three levels of master barber-surgeon according to type of examination sustained and fees paid, the lowest level

being the village barber-surgeon who took a single three-hour examination on surgical "principles", bloodletting, abscesses, wounds and
medications.[12]

The village barber-surgeon was thus a legal practitioner as distinct from many other categories of irregular ordinary healers--military
and naval doctors, veterinarians, occasional healers drawn from the
ranks of artisans and peasants as well as charitably inclined nobles and
their wives, members of clerical healing orders, male and female, such
as the brothers of the Charité hospitals, the Augustine nursing sisters
of the Hôtels-Dieu, parish *curés*, empiricks, charlatans, magical healers,
witches, and so on.

At times, the dividing line between the ordinary practitioner received by a *communauté* and these various other denizens of the Old Régime medical landscape was somewhat blurred. Thus, surgical *communautés*
also examined and certified mid-wives, bonesetters, dentists, hernia
experts, and oculists; they permitted widows of deceased masters to rent
out the "privilege" to practice legally without examination. Finally,
there were "students"--apprentices and journeymen--who might wait many
years before taking their qualifying examinations, if they ever did.
All these persons might and presumably often did evade the *communauté's*
licensing and invade its exclusive jurisdiction over practice. But, in
principle, they belonged, however tenuously, to a legally constituted
hierarchical framework of ordinary practitioners and, together with the
master barber-surgeons, their numbers were vast.

B. Numerical Strength and Population Density

Eighteenth-century commentators guessed that there were as many as
30-40,000 barber-surgeons in the kingdom, a figure which would mean well
in excess of 1 per 1,000 inhabitants.[13] Using medical surveys from the
1780s, Jean-Pierre Goubert has found somewhat lower densities in six
northern *généralités* of France (ranging from 6.82 per 10,000 (Amiens) to
1.76 per 10,000 (Rennes)).[14]

In certain regions of the south-west of the kingdom, however, higher densities seem to have prevailed. Languedoc, the French Basque country, and the dioceses of Toulouse, Bordeaux, and probably Auch-en-
Gascogne, all had surgical densities of the order of 1 per 1,000 if we
can trust contemporary counts of surgeons and of population.[15] Even
though the data lack precision, it is clear that one is dealing with impressive proportions of ordinary practitioners.

Second, in comparison with the barber-surgeons, the number of medical doctors was minuscule. The six northern *généralités* contained fewer than 500 physicians (less than 1 per 10,000) or 1 for each 4.8 surgeons; the diocese of Toulouse (not including the city) had 101 surgeons, 134 midwives, and only 8 physicians serving a population of about 80,000.[16]

C. Geographical Distribution

If the small towns and countryside of eighteenth-century France tended to be "medical deserts," as far as physicians were concerned, barber-surgeons did not neglect small population centers. In the countryside around Toulouse, one-quarter of the villages had resident surgeons. But 95% of these tiny settlements were within 1 *lieu* (about 4 kilometers) of a practitioner, an easy walk for the surgeon at any rate.[17] The tendency of surgeons to be distributed widely throughout an overwhelmingly rural population was remarked by the lieutenant of the *communauté* at Saint-Gaudens (Haute-Garonne) in 1790; "...one can easily count one surgeon in each *bourg* or hamlet, and there are even quite tiny villages with as many as three."[18] Tours had 19 town surgeons, but more than 100 scattered through its region; tiny St. Pierre-le-Moutier (Nièvre) (population less than 2,000) counted about 120 surgeons in smaller places in its region.[19]

Of the nearly 400 surgical communities in the kingdom, almost half were located in towns with fewer than 4,000 inhabitants.[20] Between 1766 and 1789, the *communauté* at Auch (population 6,000) received more than 200 surgeons, of whom about 70% took only the single examination for village practice (the remainder, except for 5 who qualified for Auch itself, practiced in small towns in the region).[21]

D. Social Origins and Status

The ordinary practitioners in the barber-surgeon's communities came from humble social origins. This could hardly be otherwise in an early modern society in which the bourgeoisie composed less than 10% of the population.[22] A considerable amount of qualitative evidence such as legal codes, social and financial privileges, and the like indicates that physicians, as individuals and in terms of their corporate identity with the university, fell within the ranks of this privileged bourgeoisie. Surgical communities, on the other hand, were classed with *arts et métiers*, or "mechanical" professions, or, as the upper-level surgeons themselves lamented, with the "vile" occupations, because of the conjunction between barber's and surgeon's work.[23]

It is somewhat more difficult to get systematic empirical evidence on the family origins of ordinary practitioners. If one seeks to determine fathers' occupations and is fortunate enough to find such information, one then encounters the problem that a substantial proportion, if not most, ordinary practitioners were sons and often grandsons of ordinary practitioners. This does suggest a traditional artisanal occupation with little upward social mobility, but it remains difficult to locate barber-surgeons in terms of other craftsmen. Among the master barber-surgeons from the diocese of Auch-en-Gascogne whom I am currently studying, at least one-third were sons of surgeons; only 4 other fathers' occupations have been found so far--2 merchants, 1 tailor, and 1 brewer.[24] Significantly, in one instance of middle-class professional background, a son and brother of notaries, who apprenticed to a village barber-surgeon in the mid-seventeenth century, the contract itself explained that the young man was in dire circumstances having lost both parents and wishing "prendre quelque mestié pour à l'avenir gagner sa pauvre vie."[25]

It seems safe to conclude that barber-surgeons came from the common people. In a predominantly peasant society, ordinary practitioners probably resembled their clients, like the surgeon in Diderot's *Jacques le Fataliste* whom the author describes as an *espèce de paysan*.[26] The Paris surgical elite recognized that the bonding their humble colleagues had with patients of similarly modest status constituted one of the strengths of the profession and a distinct market-place advantage over doctors of medicine. A memoir dated 1749 in behalf of Louis XV's *premier chirurgien*, La Martinière, remarked that the common people [*le menu peuple*] were accustomed to surgeons. Even something as apparently as trivial and irrelevant as style of dress could enter into the relationship, for the poor tended to be intimidated by physicians' attire. Common folk, of course, had a higher risk of accidents requiring surgical care as they worked at dangerous occupations.[27] Thus the specific kinds of tasks they did as well as their general style of work and life linked ordinary practitioners and manual workers. As craftsmen, however skilled, the ordinary practitioners' goals in their work (and the expectations of their clients) would have been limited to the performance of the job at hand, not to the cultivation of new knowledge.

E. Training and Careers

After completion of formal legal apprenticeship, a requirement for surgeons until the 1770s, the apprenticeship model characterized all further training of ordinary practitioners. That is, training was some-thing arranged between private individuals; recipients came away with testimonials certifying satisfactory completion of the terms of service. The particular setting might be continued service under a master in private practice as a journeyman, or military or naval service, or hos-pital experience, but the pattern was basically the same. Masters eval-uated apprentices according to their *vie et moeurs*, social and moral criteria. Diligence, attention to duty, obedience, devotion, fidelity, reliability, and other virtues counted more than merit, intelligence, talent, or skill, the latter qualities seldom receiving mention in the masters' certificates.[28] Even the surgical colleges or schools, which began to supersede apprenticeship for theoretical instruction in eighteenth-century Paris and in major provincial centers, did not make an evaluation of ability in cognitive matters; they too issued certifi-cates of attendance rather than grades. Surgical schools did not have admission requirements, nor the power to grant degrees or licenses to practice.[29]

Licensing remained a regional matter under the control of the local *communautés*. If we can take Auch-en-Gascogne once again as typical of a traditional surgical *communauté*, virtually all who became master sur-geons were natives of the diocese, and more than one-half qualified for practice in the same village or town in which they had been born. Of-ten, home-town practice meant a return to rather than a failure to leave one's birthplace, for ordinary practitioners displayed remarkable geo-graphical mobility. Like other artisans, barber-surgeons evidently par-ticipated in elaborate *tours de France* lasting many years and usually including a period in Paris.[30] At Auch, (where about 30% of the masters had studied at Paris) the age of reception to the mastership tended to be advanced, averaging nearly 40 years, and varied greatly. About as many became masters in their fifties as in their twenties.[31]

F. Practice

The ordinary practitioner engaged in every kind of medical activity as well as other kinds of work no longer recognized today as part of medicine. In eighteenth-century France, cutting hair and trimming beards remained central to the livelihood of ordinary practitioners, especially during the long and mobile period before they became masters, if they ever did.[32]

Pharmacy and treatment of internal ailments, though legally prohibited to barber-surgeons, also entered into their practice in a major way. My claim here is not that barber-surgeons had the training, knowledge, or therapeutic skills to deal with medical problems as well as physicians of the time; contemporaries, especially those concerned with medical reform, loudly and perhaps somewhat hastily condemned ordinary practitioners as incompetent and dangerous. Even a surgical lieutenant complained that most country practitioners knew only how to shave and bleed.[33] The fact remains, however, that those affiliated with surgical communities must have had a broad market for their services or they would not have maintained such numbers. That they rather than medical doctors served as ordinary practitioners was obviously the case throughout most of eighteenth-century France where, as we have seen, physicians were absent or very few.

The same pattern obtained in the major cities too: at Paris a leading physician of the medical Faculty admitted that the sick consulted first with surgeons; surgeons themselves noted: "The *fauxbourgs* of Paris, refuges of the poor citizenry, contain more people than a good many major cities of the kingdom; yet no physicians live in the *fauxbourgs*."[34] The conclusion appeared obvious: "[the surgeon] will always be the physician for the poor."[35] At Lyon, France's second city, a doctor of medicine estimated that surgeons (of whom there were about 100 compared with 30 physicians) pocketed 90% of the revenues from general medical practice. A state of affairs he called "medical anarchy" reigned throughout France, in cities as in the countryside.[36]

G. Relationship with the Medical Profession

Eighteenth-century surgeons thus constituted an organized group of ordinary practitioners separate and distinct from the medical profession proper. Geographical, economic, social, and cultural distance between the two groups led to de facto autonomy for ordinary practitioners, an autonomy partially recognized in law by an independent corporative structure. Despite a formal hierarchy favoring physicians, interaction between the two corporations was normally slight. In cities, however, where doctors and surgeons lived and practiced in close proximity and

where their prospective clientele might overlap, there was increased
potential for competition and conflict.

Our model of the ordinary practitioner in eighteenth-century France
has thus far presented a static picture in order to draw attention to
certain structural and fairly stable elements. The surgical profession,
in fact, experienced considerable change during this period. Although
we do not need to take up this dynamic process in detail here, a few
generalizations will help place the last two elements of the model of
the ordinary practitioner (relationship to the medical profession and
relationship to patients) in historical context.[37]

During the seventeenth and early eighteenth centuries, an elite
group of Paris surgeons cultivated a special relationship with the
French Crown. By means of royal patronage and legislation in their behalf, they modified the organization of local surgical communities so
that instead of being isolated units, the communities became an inter-
connected if somewhat loosely unified professional network. The Paris
leadership imposed on this structure new institutions in the form of a
school (1724) and an Academy (1731), both of which were royal foundations, national in scope, and centralized at Paris. A concerted effort
was undertaken to define and achieve higher educational standards and
loftier social and intellectual aspirations.

This campaign implied changes in professional relationships with
physicians, on the one hand, and the vast rank and file of barber-surgeons, on the other. Events reached a climax in April, 1743, when the
Paris surgeons secured a royal declaration requiring a university arts
degree for all Paris master surgeons and forbidding them to work as
barber-surgeons. Although the declaration of 1743 appeared to split
surgical élites from ordinary practitioners, it in fact demonstrated the
power of the Paris elite to improve the image of surgery as an occupation without surrendering any of its authority over and increasing control of ordinary practitioners throughout the kingdom.

By the 1740s, it was becoming evident to the enlightened public as
well as to an alarmed Paris medical Faculty that the surgical elite was
making good claims to professional authority over ordinary practitioners. At the same time the scientific authority of surgery was bolstered
by the publication of the first volume of *Mémoires* of the Academy of
Surgery in March, 1743. Both, of course, were domains in which medical
doctors traditionally had asserted their own prerogatives and claims to
superiority. Although physicians' interests tended to be confined to a

kind of symbolic control, this at least had never been seriously challenged. Now, as if to add insult to injury, the Paris surgeons openly
rejected symbolic deference to the medical Faculty, refusing oaths of
homage and financial tributes. Finally, the surgeons suspended recep-
tions to the mastership rather than have medical doctors continue to
preside over examination of candidates.

The mounting intraprofessional tensions boiled over into open warfare. Legal memoirs, public letters, anonymous pamphlets, broadsides,
and other literary genres were the weapons with which one side did
battle with the other.[38] Known collectively as *contestations*, because
of the legal contest over the 1743 declaration at issue, the public debate between physicians and surgeons raged from 1743 until mid-century
when the Crown intervened with compromise legislation effectively resolving the dispute in the surgeons' favor.

The *contestations* brought out into the open latent competition,
indeed hostility, between physicians and surgeons not simply or necessarily as individual practitioners, but as rival corporations. The
group representing ordinary practitioners prevailed in a legal confrontation with the officially recognized medical elite. That surgeons
rather than physicians took care of ordinary medical practice and ought
to do so had been an underlying theme in the surgeons' polemic with the
Faculty:

> this custom [of surgeons working as ordinary practi-
> tioners] is so simple, so natural, and so invariably
> established by necessity, that one could not possibly
> conceive of another more appropriate to the condition
> [l'état] of the patients and which would assure them
> with such certainty the minor aid that they receive.[39]

Victory in the *contestations* appeared to vindicate the surgeons' account
of the ordinary practitioner's role and to justify their normative conclusion that medical practice ought to be left in his hands: "the
natural order is so clearly manifested in this practice that humanity
should respect it, maintain it, and promote it by all necessary
means...."[40]

François Quesnay (1694-1774), the author of the anonymous essay of
1748 whose Enlightenment rhetoric we have just quoted, was the surgeons'
chief spokesman in the *contestations*. A clever accoucheur and surgeon,
professor of therapy at the surgical school and secretary of the Academy
of Surgery, Quesnay became physician to Louis XV's mistress, Mme de
Pompadour, and founder of the Physiocratic school of political economy.
In 1748 at the height of the *contestations* and a turning point in his

own career away from medicine, Quesnay offered his brilliant intellect and polemical skills one last time to the surgical professional cause he had served for twenty years. His *Essai impartial des Contestations des Médecins et des Chirurgiens considérées par rapport à l'intérêt Public* brought out in bold relief the last aspect of our model of the ordinary practitioner--his relationship to his patient.

According to Quesnay, it did not really matter much from a medical point of view whether physicians or surgeons treated most patients.[41] For ordinary patients typically needed only simple ("and perhaps the best") remedies: "bloodletting, *tisanne*, a few purgatives and very few other remedies."[42] What did matter was that the patient be free to choose his surgeon or physician or both. Neither medical profession should be allowed to have the power (*le pouvoir des Médecins et des Chirurgiens*) to infringe upon the patient's rights (*les droits des malades*).[43]

In most cases surgeons were chosen for the following reasons: (1) technical: competence to carry out phlebotomy, the central thera- peutic act in medicine; it was axiomatic for Quesnay that he who con- trolled phlebotomy would control ordinary practice;[44] (2) economic: surgeons cost less than physicians; they charged only for their services and materials, not for the act of consultation and advice;[45] (3) social and cultural: surgeons were more accessible and had better rapport with ordinary patients. In fact, physicians, in characterizing and carica- turing their rivals as ignorant artisans, drew attention to this social fit between surgeons and lowly patients. Surgeons, upon entering a noble household, loved to resume acquaintances with the domestics; these "lackeys" were their "old comrades": "they drink together, shake each other's hand, and slap one another on the back in a friendly way."[46]

If these considerations made surgeons the "natural" healers of the poor, ultimate power rested with the patient: "the patient alone has the absolute right to decide [on treatment] or to determine as he sees fit after having taken their [the doctor's and surgeon's] advice."[47] Wealthy patients could avail themselves of the luxury of consulting both a physician and a surgeon, but this was clearly out of the question for "nearly all men not well off,"[48] for the "poor citizens burdened with the painstaking work of society."[49]

Quesnay's analysis reflected an ancient tradition going back to Hippocratic medicine, in which the medical man's role was that of ad- viser, not arbiter or judge: "He gives advice, counsel, prescriptions,

not orders nor commands."[50] The patient remained the best judge of his
ailment as well as the life circumstances which contributed to it and
would govern its management.[51]

Also, except for the occasional charitable gesture, which by definition did not involve fees, the medical man seldom dealt with patients
of the lower social orders. He served his social equals or superiors.
It would simply not do for such a practitioner to go beyond gentle
recommendations to a patient who was at the same time a patron, and who
usually had a good understanding of theoretical medical knowledge himself. These basic intellectual and social conditions of medical practice had not changed substantially in the eighteenth century.[52] In the
doctor-patient relationship, ultimate authority belonged to the latter.

Quesnay's analysis, of course, despite the author's disingenuous
claim of impartiality, was also a shrewd tactic in the surgeons' struggle for equality with physicians. If a physician prescribed a phlebotomy for a medical condition, but both the patient and the surgeon-
phlebotomist disagreed with this choice of therapy, Quesnay declared,
the surgeon was justified in refusing to perform bloodletting.[53] Because the patient, not the physician, controlled the medical transaction, the physician should not control the surgeon either: "the physician does not have the right to order the execution of what he advises,
nor to decide the fate of patients according to his ideas." The analogy
of the physician as architect and the surgeon as mason, a favorite meta-
phor of physicians, broke down because the patient was not a block of
wood, but rather the "master" of the task at hand.[54] Both parties were
in principle subordinate to the patient they each sought to serve.

In such a situation, intraprofessional competition for patients,
for prestige, and for knowledge was no accident. Competition followed
as a necessary and even desirable structural feature of medical practice. Let the guilds compete in open and healthy rivalry [émulation].[55]
Let the most suitable practitioners, as determined by patients, prevail,
Quesnay declared, anticipating in this special case his general doctrine
of economic liberalism, freedom of trade, and the famous physiocratic
maxim, laissez faire, laissez passer.[56]

IV

General Practitioners

Our contention that structural differences, differences in kind,
separated the ordinary practitioner from the modern general medical
practitioner should by now be fairly clear. The G.P., unlike his traditional predecessor, does not and did not belong to a separate, autonomous profession, but to the same profession as the specialist or elite
practitioner. Despite numerical predominance in the profession until
perhaps the end of World War II, general practitioners in France (and
probably other European countries, too) never had the density in the
general population nor the relative numerical strength within the profession of the eighteenth-century barber-surgeons. The nineteenth-century French health officer [*officier de santé*], a kind of intermediate
form between barber-surgeon and modern general practitioner, makes an
interesting comparison in this connection. At their most numerous, the
officers of health constituted no more than about half of the French
medical corps; their density in the population on a national basis in
1845-1847 was just over 2 per 10,000, and in no region except Corsica
did they approach levels of one per 1,000 inhabitants. After the mid-
nineteenth century, numbers of officers of health declined sharply until
their abolition in 1893 when only about 2,000 survived, less than 10% of
the medical profession.[57]

In the 1880s, the French medical profession declined to population
densities as low as 3.3 per 10,000 (1886), a definite reduction from the
earlier nineteenth century (5.7 per 10,000 in 1844)[58] and, we have suggested, from the pluri-professional situation of the Old Regime. Other
European countries of the late nineteenth century like Germany (3.3 per
10,000 in 1885) and Austria (3.1 per 10,000 in 1889) had similarly modest doctor-to-population ratios; only in the last fifteen years of the
century did the growth of the profession in Continental European nations
begin to outstrip that of the population.[59] I am unable to verify whether there was also a prior "demedicalization" in the German-speaking
countries as in France. There was a sharp decline in medical densities
in Great Britain between mid-century and the 1880s. During the following three decades Britain maintained fairly constant and relatively high
levels of medical men (5.9 per 10,000 in 1881, 6.4 in 1911).[60]

Canada and, especially, the United States had much higher medical densities than European countries. In his famous *Report* of 1910, Abraham Flexner drew attention to this situation which clearly derived from the legions of marginal practitioners with medical degrees (whom we have called ordinary practitioners) then active and highly competitive in the United States.[61] But between 1870 and 1930, the American medical profession grew at a slower rate than the general population and five times slower than professional occupations as a whole. After reaching a peak of 17 doctors per 10,000 persons in 1900, the American profession dropped to 13 per 10,000 in 1930.[62] So, it would seem that modern medical professions in various countries have, at different times and in different ways and perhaps for different specific reasons, gone through a stage of elimination of ordinary practitioners.

General practitioners in nineteenth-century France tended to be located in larger towns and cities; a trend which accelerated in twentieth-century Western countries.[63] In other words, village barber-surgeons had no legitimate successors.

The G.P.'s social origins and status, however humble, were usually middle-class, unlike the artisan barber-surgeon.[64] Likewise, training of G.P.'s normally took place in schools, thus ensuring some minimum selection for and standardization of education. Most important, the nineteenth-century medical elite gained control over educational institutions, examining, and licensing of general practitioners (and of paramedical types like the French officers of health), though the precise scenario, timing, and degree of government involvement varied from one country to another.[65]

Although the evidence is sketchy and further empirical studies are needed, I would predict other changes in the career patterns of nineteenth-century general practitioners: less training under fathers,[66] greater homogeneity in terms of age of qualification for practice, a younger average age of qualification, and a reduced tendency to return to one's home town after studying elsewhere. But such trends toward modern professional structure remain to be documented and would probably be, in any case, relatively gradual changes from the ordinary practitioner career pattern. Similarly, one would expect to find G.P.'s less prone to engage openly in non-medical or even paramedical work and, in turn, to have and be perceived to have a higher, more uniform standard of medical competence.

Finally, and most problematic, is the question of the doctor-patient relationship. Was not the G.P., like the ordinary practitioner, still essentially an adviser who needed to cultivate with great tact, if not deference, a rapport with his client? This cannot be denied. Yet I would maintain that the social fit between doctor and patient gradually became less relevant, yielding to public respect for medical knowledge, training, and expertise--in short, to, in Peterson's phrase, medical "authority."[67] How medicine was perceived, and what people thought it could explain and do, began to assume priority over who one's doctor was in a social sense. In France, and probably in England as well, rising professional prestige evidently preceded major scientific breakthroughs such as the germ theory of disease.[68] Balzac's authoritative *médecin de campagne* evokes this new status of the general practitioner.

As medicine became largely a middle-class occupation, medical men in turn could and did, with the help of various kinds of social welfare programs (state and private health insurance), provide services to a greater range of classes. Medicine took on the form of what Terence Johnson calls a collegial profession, one characterized by considerable internal homogeneity, both social and intellectual, and a broad, socially heterogeneous demand for its services.[69]

V

Conclusion

If the above analysis is accurate, we are left with a discontinuity in the history of medical professionalization. A modern profession did not simply evolve gradually from eighteenth-century precedents; ordinary practitioners--barber-surgeons, apothecaries, feldshers, etc.--were not precursors, in any meaningful developmental sense, of general practitioners. On the contrary, ordinary practitioners declined, became extinct, and were replaced by G.P.'s just as elite physicians and surgeons of the Old Régime disappeared in favor of modern specialists.

If there was such a transformation in professional structure, what brought it about? Some causes were as general, complex, and interwoven as demographic expansion and population migration from village to town and city, the rise of well-to-do urban middle classes, industrialization, and capitalism.[70] All these acted to create a demand for and a supply of new professional men in medicine as well as in other fields that sought to satisfy material needs and secular values. Increasingly powerful centralized governments attempted (first, on an ideological level, but later by practical policies) to counter regional distinctions by establishing national patterns, standards, and goals in health as in other sensitive areas of social management. Older patterns of aristocratic and monarchical patronage declined.[71]

Factors operating within medicine are equally familiar and difficult to separate from one another. The profession's capture of hospitals and their conversion into instruments for research and teaching gave medicine something it had never had before (except perhaps in the military setting)--a specific, controlled environment as a work place. Poor patients, once viewed as clients by ordinary practitioners or as souls deserving charity by the church, became clinical material while alive and subjects for anatomical study after death. They were admitted and treated under conditions set by the profession instead of by themselves or secular authorities. This transformation, as it first occurred in Revolutionary and early nineteenth-century Paris, has been documented by Michel Foucault and Erwin Ackerknecht, each in his own quite different way.[72] Nevertheless, both authors agree on the time, place, and historic significance of the medicalization of hospitals, a process whose sociological implications Erving Goffman has discussed.[73]

I have maintained elsewhere and suggested in this paper that professional unification helped bring about a modern medical profession.[74] Specifically, the unification of medicine and surgery and the formation of unified yet specialized training institutions marked a decisive change from earlier patterns. Educational unification provided a basis for the production of highly trained, uniformly trained practitioners.[75] By placing administrative power firmly in the hands of a professional elite (with influential connections in society or directly with government), unification made it possible to impose standards and reduce intraprofessional competition. An achievement of the Revolution in France, this type of medical unification gradually emerged in England during the middle decades of the nineteenth century and still later in North America.

The rapid growth of esoteric, increasingly technical aspects of medicine no longer accessible to laymen, not even to the best educated, also contributed to professional transformation. Here we can only list the following: emerging medical sciences, the first of which was pathological anatomy; specialization; methodological innovations, in particular, the applications of statistics to public health, pathology, and therapy;

and a host of new instruments and diagnostic techniques, such as the
stethoscope for mediate ausculation. Apparently absent, however, it
should be noted, was an objective increase in therapeutic efficacy.[76]

One way to assess the impact of this bewildering array of novelties
on professional transformation is to view it in terms of power.[77] In
place of the traditional arrangement in which power rested with the
patient rather than the ordinary practitioner, the modern medical profession acquired three types of power: (1) power in society as expressed in terms of high prestige, career opportunities, social authority,
and political influence; (2) power over its own profession as expressed
by elite control and values, institutional unity, and high standards of
entry and training; and (3) power over patients.

One has only to consider the modern hospital interaction, epitomized by a surgical operation, to comprehend the extent of this third
category of power. Already in the early nineteenth century, before
anesthesia, before the aseptic operating room and the impressive symbolic as well as biological sterility of the surgeon's white gown, mask,
and rubber gloves, a radical transformation in power had taken place.
Baron Dupuytren, the Napoleon of surgery, who totally dominated and, at
times, brutalized unfortunate charity patients on his wards at the
Hôtel-Dieu of Paris during the first third of the nineteenth century,
may have been flagrant and excessive. Dupuytren, however, with his
virtues and faults, personified a new image of heroic physician.[78]

Hospital medical men, as a group, and the profession they led, made
good their claims to power over patients. More often and more subtly
expressed than the direct brutality of a Dupuytren was the physician's
calm and confident assertion that he knew the patient's illness more
accurately and intimately than did the patient himself.[79] Invoking
their newly acquired knowledge and techniques, physicians dislodged
patients from the privileged position they had held with respect to
their own bodies and ailments. This represented considerably more than
a dramatic increase in medical knowledge and technology; it was a rever-
sal in power relationships whereby physicians acquired the power to impose their professional definitions of disease. Ordinary practitioners
had never aspired to nor dreamed of such power. In this sense, the decline of the ordinary practitioner and the rise of a modern profession
were different but complementary aspects of the same transformation.

NOTES

1   Jacques Léonard, *La Vie Quotidienne du Médecin de Province au XIXe
    Siècle* (Paris: Hachette, 1977); M. Jeanne Peterson, *The Medical
    Profession in Mid-Victorian London* (Berkeley: U. of Cal. Press,
    1978).

2   Peterson cites in particular Eliot Freidson, *Profession of Medicine.
    A Study of the Sociology of Applied Knowledge* (New York, 1970) as a
    "theoretical underpinning" for her own work. Léonard's doctoral
    thesis, *Les médecins de l'ouest au XIXe siècle*, Atelier de repro-
    duction des thèses de Lille III, 3 vol. (Paris: Champion, 1978),
    reflects more fully the *Annales* methodology applied to medical his-
    tory. See also special number of *Annales ESC*, 32 (Sept.-Oct. 1977),
    "Médecins, Médecine et Société en France aux XVIIIe et XIXe siècles."

3   The expressions are from Freidson and Ivan Illich, *Medical Nemesis:
    The Expropriation of Health* (London: Calder and Boyars, 1975).

4   Ivan Waddington, "General Practitioners and Consultants in Early
    Nineteenth-Century England: The Sociology of Intra-Professional
    Conflict," in *Health Care and Popular Medicine in Nineteenth Century
    England, Essays in the Social History of Medicine*, ed. John Woodward
    and David Richards (New York, 1977), pp. 164-168, makes a similar
    point. I have discussed the specialization side of the problem in
    "The Origins of a Modern Concept of Medical Specialization: John
    Morgan's *Discourse* of 1765," *Bulletin of the History of Medicine* 50
    (1976), 511-535.

5   Léonard, *La Vie Quotidienne*, pp. 165-170; Robert Heller, *"Officiers
    de Santé*: The Second-Class Doctors of Nineteenth Century France,"
    Medical History, 22 (1978), 25-43.

6   Henry Sigerist, *Socialized Medicine in the Soviet Union* (New York,
    1937), pp. 74, 144.

7   Peterson, pp. 37-38.

8   S. W. F. Holloway, "Medical Education in England, 1830-1858: A
    Sociological Analysis," *History*, 49 (1964), 299.

9   *Ibid.*, p. 324.

10 See Terence J. Johnson, *Professions and Power* (London: Macmillan,
    1972), pp. 63-74; N. D. Jewson, "Medical Knowledge and the Patronage
    System in 18th Century England," *Sociology* 8 (1974), 369-385;
    Catherine W. Zerner, "The New Professionalism in the Renaissance,"
    in *The Architect*, ed. S. Kostof (New York, 1977), pp. 124-128.

11 For more detailed descriptions of and references to primary sources
    on the surgical *communautés*, see Toby Gelfand, "Medical Profession-
    als and Charlatans. The *Comité de Salubrité enquête* of 1790-91,"
    Histoire Sociale-Social History 11 (1978), 62-97, and Gelfand,
    "Deux cultures, une profession: Les Chirurgiens Français au XVIIIe

siècle," *Revue d'histoire moderne et contemporaine* 27 (1980), 468-484.

12 *Statuts et Règlements Généraux pour les maîtres en chirurgie des provinces du royaume*, 1730, 5th ed. (Paris, 1772), pp. 45-46.

13 C. P. Luynes, *Mémoires sur la cour de Louis XV: 1735-1768*, ed. L. Dussieux and E. Soulie (Paris, 1860-1865), vol. 1, p. 143; François Chaussier, *Mémoire sur quelques abus dans la constitution des corps et collèges de chirurgie* (Dijon, 1789), pp. 29, 32-33.

14 Jean-Pierre Goubert, "The Extent of Medical Practice in France around 1780," *Journal of Social History*, 10 (1977), 410-427.

15 Mireille Laget, "La naissance aux siècles classiques," *Annales ESC* 32 (1977), 980-984; P. Thillaud, "Les maladies et la médecine en pays basque nord à la fin de l'ancien régime," thèse de IIIème cycle, Université de Paris-I (1977), pp. 158-162; AD Hérault C 525, "Etat du nombre des médecins, chirurgiens, et sage-femmes qui sont dans les communautés du département de Toulouse (1783)"; Philippe Loupès, "L'Assistance paroissiale aux pauvres malades dans le diocèse de Bordeaux au XVIIIe siècle," *Annales du Midi* 84 (1972), 47; AD Gers E 304, "Registre des récipiendaires pour la maîtrise en l'art de chirurgie de la communauté d'Auch."

16 AD Hérault, C 525.

17 *Ibid.*

18 Archives Nationales (Paris), F17 2276, doss. 2, pièce 277; In the diocese of Bordeaux (mid-18th century), 45% of the rural parishes had at least 1 surgeon, and 10% had between 3 and 5; Loupès, p. 47.

19 Gelfand, "Medical Professionals and Charlatans," p. 95.

20 *Ibid.*, p. 97.

21 AD Gers E 304.

22 Pierre Goubert, *L'Ancien Régime 1: la Société* (Paris: Armand Colin, 1969), pp. 165-209.

23 Toby Gelfand, "From Guild to Profession: The Surgeons of France in the 18th Century," *Texas Reports on Biology and Medicine* 32 (1974), 121-134.

24 AD Gers, série 5E (registres paroissiales). In a series of 19 apprenticeship contracts involving Toulouse master surgeons between 1738 and 1772, the following occupations of apprentices' fathers are given: master wigmaker, turner, printer, town official, bourgeois, royal official, painter, messenger, 2 surgeons, and 4 *habitants*; AD Haute Garonne, E 1152, 1153. Fifty-three applications for reception by surgeons for the Bordeaux region between 1693 and 1706 mentioned 14 fathers' occupations, of which 12 surgeons, 1 wine merchant, 1 cloth merchant. AD Gironde, 6E 24.

25 Gabriel Laplagne-Barris, "Un contrat d'apprentissage de chirurgien barbier au XVIIe siècle à Montesquiou," *Bulletin de la Société*

Archéologique, Historique, Littéraire et Scientifique du Gers 80 (1979), 494-496.

26 Denis Diderot, *Oeuvres romanesques*, ed. H. Bénac (Paris: Garnier, 1962), p. 496.

27 *Mémoire présenté au Roy par son Premier Chirurgien* (Paris, 1749), pp. 38-39.

28 AD Gers, E 304.

29 Gelfand, "Deux cultures."

30 AD Gers, E 304. Information on the surgical *tour de France* is particularly rich from the Bordeaux applicants to the mastership. Virtually all claimed to have "parcouru les bonnes villes" during periods lasting on the average nearly 18 years. Of the 28 candidates who mentioned towns by name, 18 had visited Paris. Other stopping places were Lyon (7 mentions), Nantes (6), Toulouse (6), La Rochelle (5) and Montpellier (3). AD Gironde, 6E 24.

31 AD Gers, E 304. The pattern was similar at Bordeaux. AD Gironde, 6E 24.

32 Gelfand, "Deux cultures."

33 Gelfand, "Medical Professionals and Charlatans," esp. pp. 74-75.

34 *Mémoire présenté au Roy par son Premier Chirurgien* (Paris, (1749), p. 37; E.-C. Bourru, *Discours prononcé aux écoles de médecine* (Paris, 1780), p. 20. Another spokesman for the surgeons claimed that common working people living in the center of Paris (les domestiques, les compagnons ouvriers, et les autres artisans, bornés à un médiocre salaire) likewise could not "hope" for care from physicians. [François Quesnay], *Examen impartial des Contestations des Médecins et des Chirurgiens, considérées par rapport à l'intérêt public* (Paris, 1748), p. 73.

35 *Mémoire présenté au Roy*, p. 39.

36 Jean-Emmanuel Gilibert, *L'anarchie médicinale ou la médecine considérée comme nuisible à la société* (Neufchâtel, 1772), vol. 1, p. 357.

37 The following discussion is based on my *Professionalizing Modern Medicine: Paris Surgeons and Medical Science and Institutions in the Eighteenth Century* (Westport, Connecticut: Greenwood Press, 1980), esp. chapter 4.

38 A. Pauly, *Bibliographie des Sciences Médicales* (London, 1954), 677-694 lists 102 printed items under the heading "Contestations relatives à la Déclaration du Roi du 23 avril 1743."

39 [François Quesnay], *Examen Impartial des Contestations des Médecins et de Chirurgiens, considérées par rapport à l'intérêt Public* (Paris, 1748), p. 75.

40 *Ibid.*

41 *Ibid.*, pp. 52-53, 58-59.

42 *Ibid.*, p. 71.

43 *Ibid.*, p. 52.

44 *Ibid.*, pp. 84-85, 122-123. "L'exercice de la Médecine chez le menu peuple est attaché à la saignée." Quesnay pointed out as well that bloodletting had crucial economic importance for surgical training and for the mobility and sustenance of young surgeons: "Or, c'est principalement pour les aider à pratiquer la saignée que les Maîtres ont chez eux des Elèves, qu'ils payent, et qu'ils nourrissent. Ils ont donc intérêt qu'ils les dédommagent de ces frais, par le lucre même que leurs procurent les saignées.... C'est la saignée qui procure aux Elèves en Chirurgie la facilité de venir de toutes les Provinces du Royaume, à Paris...ils peuvent se soutenir sans frais à Paris, jusqu'à ce qu'ils soient capables de former un établissement."

45 *Ibid.*, pp. 66, 71-72. "Les Chirurgiens font les saignées qui leur sont payées à bas prix: Et par-dessus le marché, ils conseillent le reste, en sorte que les pauvres malades sont secourus gratuitement, en ce qui concerne les fonctions qui sont du ressort de la profession du Médecin."

46 *Le Médecin véridique à l'Avocat curieux* (La Haye, 1747), p. 40.

47 Quesnay, *Examen Impartial*, p. 98.

48 *Ibid.*, pp. 63, 72.

49 *Ibid.*, pp. 75-76.

50 *Ibid.*, p. 140. For the doctor-patient relationship in Greek antiquity, see *Ancient Medicine. Selected Papers of Ludwig Edelstein*, ed. O. and C. L. Temkin (Baltimore: Johns Hopkins Press, 1967), esp. "Hippocratic Prognosis," pp. 87-110, and "The Relation of Ancient Philosophy to Medicine," pp. 349-366.

51 See William Coleman, "Health and Hygiene in the Encyclopédie: A Medical Doctrine for the Bourgeoisie," *Journal of the History of Medicine* 29 (1974), 399-421, esp. 402-406 in which the individual's primary responsibility for his own health is discussed in the context of the ancient doctrines of the "non-naturals" (environmental factors) and the healing power of nature. Coleman describes the physician's role as "that of pedagogue and advocate."

52 *Ibid.*, Jewson, "Medical Knowledge."

53 Quesnay, *Examen Impartial*, pp. 145-149.

54 *Ibid.*, pp. 138-141. "...il n'y a qu'eux [les malades] qui ont le droit d'ordonner au Chirurgien...."

55 *Ibid.*, p. 80. "L'émulation entre deux Corps également capables de cultiver la Science de l'Art de Guérir, assurait aux Citoyens des Hommes supérieurs dans la Médecine et dans la Chirurgie." See also pp. 52-53.

56 The medical sources of Quesnay's concept of economic liberalism re-
    main to be explored. For a recent general discussion see Elizabeth
    Fox-Genovese, *The Origins of Physiocracy: Economic Revolution and
    Social Order in Eighteenth-Century France* (Ithaca, N. Y.: Cornell
    U.P., 1976).

57 Léonard, pp. 166-170, George Sussman, "The Glut of Doctors in Mid-
    Nineteenth Century France," *Comparative Studies in Society and
    History*, 19 (1977), 287-304.

58 Léonard, pp. 47-51, 173-176.

59 Abraham Flexner, *Medical Education in Europe* (New York, 1912), pp.
    16-31.

60 *Ibid.*, p. 29; W. J. Reader, *Professional Men. The Rise of the Pro-
    fessional Classes in Nineteenth-Century England* (London: Weidenfeld
    and Nicolson, 1966), pp. 208-211. During the decade 1851-1861, the
    medical profession (physicians and surgeons) decreased by 18% while
    the population of England and Wales increased by 12%. For the per-
    iod 1841-1881, the figures were -14% and +63.2% respectively.

61 Abraham Flexner, *Medical Education in the United States and Canada*
    (New York, Carnegie Foundation Bulletin no. 4, 1910), pp. 14-19;
    Jacques Bernier, "Les praticiens de la santé au Québec, 1871-1921:
    Quelques données statistiques," *Recherches sociographiques* 20
    (1979), 41-58.

62 H. Dewey Anderson and Percy E. Davidson, *Occupational Trends in the
    United States* (Stanford U. Press, 194), pp. 494-497, 534-540.

63 Léonard, pp. 8-9; Flexner.

64 Léonard, esp. pp. 13-51; Peterson *passim*, esp. pp. 194-204.

65 Peterson, pp. 37, 88-89, 241-243; George Weisz, "The Politics of
    Medical Professionalization in France 1845-1848," *Journal of Social
    History* 10 (1977), 3-30, esp. 4.

66 The father-son pattern nevertheless remained common. See Peterson,
    pp. 41-44; Léonard, pp. 14-18.

67 Peterson, pp. 283-287.

68 *Ibid.*, pp. 3-4; Léonard, pp. 252-254.

69 Johnson, pp. 51-54.

70 Magali S. Larson, *The Rise of Professionalism* (Berkeley: U. of Cal.
    Press, 1977) presents a compelling analysis in terms of the "great
    transformation" to industrial capitalism. The expression is Karl
    Polanyi's. See esp. pp. 2, 9, 76-80.

71 Norbert Elias, *La Société de Cour*, trad. P. Kamnitzer (Paris: Cal-
    man-Levy, 1974); Michel de Certeau, Dominique Julia, Jacques Revel,
    *Une politique de la langue: la Révolution Française et les patois:
    l'enquête de Grégoire* (Paris: Galimard, 1975).

72 Michel Foucault, *Naissance de la Clinique*, 2d ed. (Paris: P.U.F.,
    1972); Erwin H. Ackerknecht, *Medicine at the Paris Hospital 1794-
    1848* (Baltimore: Johns Hopkins University Press, 1967).

73 Erving Goffman, "The Medical Model and Mental Hospitalization: Some
    Notes on the Vicissitudes of the Tinkering Trades," in *Asylums.
    Essays on the social situation of mental patients and other inmates*
    (Garden City, N.Y.: Anchor, 1961), pp. 321-386. See also Ivan
    Waddington, "The Role of the Hospital in the Development of Modern
    Medicine: A Sociological Analysis," *Sociology* 7 (1973), 211-225.

74 Gelfand, *Professionalizing Modern Medicine*.

75 Larson, p. 31.

76 Ackerknecht, esp. pp. 129-138.

77 Johnson; N. D. Jewson, "The Disappearance of the Sick Man From Medi-
    cal Cosmology, 1770-1870," *Sociology* 10 (1976), 225-244.

78 *The Parisian Education of An American Surgeon. Letters of Jonathan
    Mason Warren (1832-1835)*, ed. Russell M. Jones (Philadelphia:
    American Philosophical Society, 1978), pp. 108, 189. With private
    patients, however, Dupuytren was "another man." Other leading
    clinicians exhibited similar, if less extreme, behavior toward ward
    patients. *Ibid.*, pp. 116-229.

79 See Georges Canguilhem, *Le normal et le pathologique*, 2d ed. (Paris:
    P.U.F., 1972), pp. 50-51. Canguilhem cites the example of patients'
    mistaken references of pain to immediately underlying organs, as in
    "kidney pain." Modern clinicians, he concludes, are led "...à tenir
    l'expérience pathologique directe du patient comme négligeable,
    voire même comme systématiquement falsificatrice du fait patholo-
    gique objectif."

HEALTH CULTURES

IN

CONFLICT

DOMINANCE AND DOMINATION IN HEALTH CARE:
A TRANSCULTURAL PERSPECTIVE

HAZEL H. WEIDMAN

Complex historical forces have brought us to the point of questioning the power and authority of our dominant health institutions. There
is no way to describe these forces in a short paper. In my view, however, four important evolutionary processes have helped to generate
some of the ethical issues before us. These are: (a) global population
shifts; (b) rapidly expanding biomedical knowledge; (c) technological
advancements in biomedical engineering; and (d) continuing growth and
differentiation of the organizational structure which supports the
health-care enterprise. All have economic implications which have their
own impact, and together they have tended to encourage the transformation of dominance and authority in health care into something akin to
domination and arbitrary rule.

The means whereby such a transformation is achieved may lie in the
degree of alienation experienced by both providers and consumers as a
consequence of functional divisions into separate moral communities,
one being that of the medically and scientifically "informed"; the
other being that of the medically and scientifically "uninformed." A
by-product of the above trends is that more and more individuals fall
into the medically "uninformed" category.

Not only do cultural differences in health beliefs and practices
work toward increased distance and failures of communication between
health providers and consumers; so, also, do the differences in levels
of biomedical knowledge. In addition, there are great gaps in technical
information related to computerized medicine, implantable devices, and
electromechanical prostheses, all a part of the growing field of biomedical engineering, to say nothing of the field of genetic engineering.
These all add to the problem of differences between the conceptual and
ethical worlds of providers and consumers. The economics of medical
care and the value of the physician's time may represent other alienating factors as the length of time shrinks that can be allotted to doctor-patient contact. The very size and complexity of many health facilities contribute in their own intimidating ways to the functional

separation of insiders and outsiders, the medically informed and the
medically uninformed.

From these alienating processes come the large questions regarding
patient rights: "Whose life is it, anyway?"; regarding community
rights: "Why do you impose your ways upon us?"; "Why don't you respond
to our needs?"; and regarding medical ethics: "Wherein lies moral authority?" These and many other questions reflect a growing concern
about the uses of medical authority which increasingly seem linked to
absolute and arbitrary value positions.

Population shifts, growing bodies of knowledge, advancing technologies, and highly elaborated social structures would not necessarily reinforce the separation of the "informed" and the "uninformed" were it
not for some of the premises that undergird the health care system.
The orthodox social institution called "modern medicine" has emerged
from a technological, social, and political process that places a high
value upon science, professionalism, and technological achievements. At
the heart of that system, which has been sanctioned as being responsible
for the health of national populations in the industrialized areas of
the world, there is an assumption which may be eliciting some of our
current questions about power and authority in medical care. The assumption is that, "Only scientific knowledge is valid insofar as matters
of health and illness are concerned." Some of the epistemological consequences of that premise might be expressed as a logical proposition
such as the following:

> Only scientific knowledge is valid insofar as
> matters of health are concerned. I (as a mem-
> ber of the orthodox health profession) have
> scientific knowledge; therefore, I have know-
> ledge. You (all of you others outside the
> modern health profession) have no scientific
> knowledge; therefore, you have no knowledge.[1]

If we relate the historical processes outlined above to this type
of logical proposition, it is easy to see why there is a growing concern
about the uses of medical authority. Its premises are not in accord
with reality from the point of view of other cultures, other disciplines,
and various individuals who are the recipients of orthodox care. Although there are some who do not, many orthodox health professional accept such assumptions and act on them. They may do so subconsciously,
without self-awareness, but because they do, they in effect establish
their own moral universe. This moral universe is supported and enhanced
by every new medically related scientific discovery, every new medical
technological development, every new biomedical theory, and every new

edifice constructed to support such advancement. Furthermore, the boundaries of this growing medico-industrial organization are more sharply
defined by every new cultural group whose premises about health knowledge may not be compatible with those of scientific medicine. Although
not explicitly stated, many of the issues under discussion during this
conference are intimately bound to these cultural, informational technological, and social organizational processes that function *systemically*
to help transform the dominant health institution into a dominating
one.

     "Dominance" is a relatively neutral term describing a state of con-
sensually validated authority, but "domination" carries a very different
connotation which includes the exercise of arbitrary or overbearing
rule--which is the equivalent of tyrannizing over some individual or
group. It is easy to understand why "dominance" applies to orthodox
processes of health care in the contemporary world. The orthodox system
has been legitimized as *the* responsible institution. But to what extent
is "domination" applicable? How could anyone involved in the humane
task of preventing illness, maintaining health, and restoring sick individuals to an improved health status be viewed as "tyrannizing" over
anyone? The matter becomes clearer if we shift from a unicultural to a
transcultural perspective. In what follows I shall be focusing upon
only one of the factors mentioned above as contributing importantly to
the transformation of a dominant institution into a dominating one;
namely, cultural factors in health care that are linked to population
shifts.

     In the contemporary world there is no way to disregard unprecedent-
ed population shifts and migrations from one nation to another and from
rural areas into the urban centers of the world: East and West Indians
into Britain, Indonesians into Holland, Cambodians into Thailand, Viet-
namese into the United States and other countries of the world, Afghans
into Pakistan, Pakistanis into Canada, more than half a million Cubans
into Florida within the past twenty years and anywhere from 1000 to
5000 per week pouring into Key West in May, 1980. Within a month's time
the United States Cuban population alone has grown by 60,000, and many
of these people are being relocated to regions of the country where
there may or may not already be large Spanish-speaking groups. Global-
ly, these migration patterns have established in the contemporary world
two overarching social facts: (1) the populations for which national
governments and their human service programs are responsible are now

multicultural in character; (2) the institutions serving these multicultural populations remain unicultural in design, substance, and mission. Some of our central problems in health care relate to these
facts.

In this era of mass movement and reshaping of social, political,
and economic structures, it has been brought home to us that human service programs, including medical care, are not uniformly applicable--as
we at one time thought they were. We have found that they are not
equally supportive of all groups; not equally security-enhancing, equally restorative, or equally responsive to culturally influenced human
needs.

Our institutional forms, which we define as needing some modification, perhaps, but as being essentially sound and appropriate, at one
time may have been admirably suited to the populace from which they
emerged and for which they were designed. Subsequent groups which have
come to our countries, however, have felt the impact of these institutions and been alienated by them even as they have been supported by
them. Some aspects of the problem are sketched below.

Every social group described and studied, whether from archaeologi-
cal evidence, historical record, or direct observation, has been shown
to hold dear its own pharmacopeias and therapeutic paradigms, its own
beliefs and practices about health maintenance and cure. Furthermore,
every society recognizes healing specialists who provide health care to
members of the group. True, scientific methods and knowledge are not
central in these health cultural traditions; nevertheless, the traditions themselves are viewed as meaningful and valid, and they are as
intrinsic to the overall cultural configuration of each society as orthodox medicine has been an integral part of the Western cultural experience.

When immigrants into host countries leave their places of origin,
they bring with them their traditional ways of coping, of maintaining
health and a sense of well-being, and of treating illness. When there
are sufficient numbers of them in a particular locality, they do this in
traditional ways within their own social networks and institutional
structures despite the acculturative pressures upon them.

Successful adaptation of the immigrants to the social, political,
and economic spheres of activity in a new nation requires the denial,
repression, or lack of use of traditional models in favor of those of
the host country. This is not an easy transition to make, and in the

acculturative processes experienced by all immigrant groups, there is a
fundamental inequity and process of dehumanization. Host cultures are
comprised of institutions and patterns of behavior that are viewed from
unicultural perspectives as being "good" and "right" and "best." This
means that all other cultural beliefs and behaviors that do not match
relatively well the organizational principles and social forms of the
host culture, are viewed as something less than desirable. Members of
every incoming group have felt the impact of intolerance for their own
cultural styles and have experienced debasement because of it. In many
ways the trauma is unavoidable, becaue it is inherent in most interactions they have with members of the host country. This creates problems of adaptation in all spheres of activity in the new cultural setting. Some of these are explored below as we focus on such problems in
health care.

From a transcultural perspective it is important to note that aspects of immigrant groups' cultural traditions are organized into health
cultures[2]--systems similar to the health culture of orthodox medicine in
structure and purpose but dissimilar in health beliefs, customary health
behaviors, and accepted treatments.[3] Although newcomers may utilize
orthodox health facilities, they cannot shed automatically their security-enhancing traditional approaches to health and illness. They retain
them and utilize them in their efforts toward health. All too often,
however, the health cultural beliefs of patients are viewed by orthodox
providers of care as irrational or superstitious, negative, and as a
symptom of ignorance. They are, therefore, not taken into account in
diagnosis and treatment.

The problem of traditional health culture versus the health culture
of orthodox medicine assumes particular significance in urban settings
containing multiethnic (multicultural) populations. It is here that the
traditional health cultures flourish, because they are reinforced by new
immigrants and by the security of individuals living among cultural peers.
In fact, a substantial portion of health care in such communities is provided through traditional means, including self-treatment and family care
according to tenets of the local health culture and the services of the
traditional healers. It is not uncommon for individuals to seek help
simultaneously from both the traditional health care system and that of
orthodox medicine. From an organizational point of view these may be
described as "competing" systems--but not from an individual recipient's
point of view.

The existence of traditional health cultures is generally unrecog-
nized or ignored by orthodox health practitioners. Usually they are not
trained to be aware of them and may even be taught to deny the possibility of their significance if they are acknowledged. Because of the assumptions described earlier, the orthodox practitioner tends subconsciously to operate as if his or her diagnosis and treatment provided
the only correct assessment of the situation. He or she tends, also,
to assume that the patient concurs and is anxious to comply in order to
be cured. Understandably, in the light of assumptions regarding the
validity of only scientific knowledge, the patient's beliefs about symptoms, about illness, about bodily functioning, maintenance of health,
and recovery of health are too often disregarded. At the least this im-
poses upon an individual a sense of lowered worth; at the worst, significant misunderstandings arise between orthodox health professionals and
the patients they serve. One possible result of such misunderstandings
may be that the patient is concerned about an entirely different kind of
process (culturally or *emically* defined condition)[4] from that which has
caught the attention of the practitioner (medically or *etically*-defined
condition).[5] The practitioner may then proceed to treat the patient in
ways which the patient views as totally inappropriate. The Haitian
syndrome of *battement de coeur*[6] is a case in point.

> The basis set of symptoms consists of pain all
> over the body, sleeplessness, and an unpredictably but
> wildly beating heart. *Battement de coeur* is perceived
> to be a very serious condition--so serious in fact that
> some Haitians showing symptoms of the condition express
> a desire to return to Haiti to die. When they present
> their symptoms to physicians...they are examined care-
> fully. Then they tend to be released under tranquili-
> zing medication or with a prescription for such medi-
> cation. They are, in a sense, patted on the head, re-
> assured that there is nothing seriously wrong, that
> the condition is self-limiting, and are sent home with
> a medical diagnosis of "stress reaction; paroxysmal
> tachycardia".
> The diagnosis of stress reaction may make unques-
> tionably good sense in our terms. The medical findings
> justify it. The particular nature of the acculturation
> problem for Haitians in Miami supports it. Neverthe-
> less, the patient leaves feeling that the physician
> has not recognized his real problem or dealt with it
> in any way. In his eyes, the condition is caused by
> an insufficient supply of blood. He believes that he
> literally does not have enough blood in his body for
> his heart to distribute it easily. Not only is there
> too little blood, it is also perceived to be weakened
> blood, that is, pinkish and mucous-like rather than
> good red blood.

> Consequently, the heart is perceived to beat
> wildly, because it must work so hard to circu-
> late an insufficient and nutritionally inade-
> quate supply of blood throughout the body.
> Appropriate therapy in the patient's eyes
> would be some sort of blood tonic such as *eau
> de melisse*, which is available to him in Haiti
> but not in Miami.[7]

Here we see one of the distressing outcomes of encounters guided
by a unicultural perspective. The patient's concerns are focused upon
an entirely different kind of problem from that upon which the health
professional's attention is centered. The practitioner is responding
to the same set of symptoms as the patient, but his efforts are directed toward treating and reassuring him in ways that have no meaning
for the patient. Such instances, multiplied many times in every health
context in which an ethnic patient meets an orthodox provider of care,
help get the point across to the patient that his perceptions, knowledge, and experiences have little significance for the management of
his current health problems. They reinforce the silent behavior-based
"statement" that his beliefs are not worth inquiring about, that his
own health cultural tradition is to be ignored, and that his customary
health practices are to be disregarded. How arrogant this must seem,
and how demeaning this must be to patients whose health cultural back-
grounds are non-congruent with those of the dominant system. Is this
not dehumanizing in the extreme? And when it occurs, does it not meet
the criteria for a shift from dominance to domination in health care?[8]

The exclusion of traditional health cultural beliefs and practices
from the realm of meaning and medical discourse is unnecessary, ineffi-
cient, expensive, and in some instances actually destructive. Both the
traditional and the orthodox systems, presumably, are attempting to
achieve the same result: an improved health status for the patient. It
is, therefore, quite likely that orthodox medicine will become more successful in pursuing and attaining this goal by introducing a transcultural perspective which will expand its views on health, its maintenance
and restoration. Some efforts have been made in this direction, but
there has not been sufficient general adoption of the transcultural view
to prevent many groups of people from remaining somewhat alienated from
orthodox medical practices. It is highly desirable that more orthodox
health professionals, particularly those in primary care, develop an
ability to become culturally sensitive providers, utilizing aspects of
both systems at the same time: orthodox medicine and traditional health
cultural beliefs and practices. This will allow them to assume the role

of "brokers" or cultural negotiators, mediating for the patient between
two systems so as to arrive at an acceptable clarification of the patient's problem and an acceptable treatment.

"Falling-out" can serve as a useful paradigm for the transcultural
approach to health care. Falling-out is a culturally defined (*emic*)
disorder found among Southern Black Americans, Bahamians (where it is
more often termed "blacking-out"), and Haitians (where it is called
indisposition). It expresses itself typically with symptoms of collapse and a constricted state of consciousness. The evidence compiled
to date suggests that falling-out may be a health problem with a significant prevalence.[9]

Falling-out occurs in a variety of contexts--at religious services
or funerals, during arguments, as a result of psycho-sexual conflict,
in the face of unbearable social ambiguities such as those found in
low-income inner-city areas, as a result of tension or failure in
sports--but with similar symptoms. It is viewed within the culture
(*emically*) as normal and expected behavior in many instances. However,
it is defined as a sickness when its frequency, duration, and/or unpredictability become such as to seriously interfere with normal functioning. As a sickness it may even produce a threat to life.[10]

When episodes of falling-out occur, the traditional health culture
provides a range of etiologic possibilities for the condition. Depending upon the level of analysis, these include: proximate causes
(heated, thickened, rising blood); intermediate causes (family inheri-
tance of magical harm, spirits); or ultimate causes (God, enemies).
Appropriate remedies are utilized for whatever cause is distinguished
at a particular time.

The orthodox practitioner who is presented with the symptoms or
even a chief complaint of falling-out, usually makes diagnoses based
upon an outside (*etic*) view of the problem. Sometimes the symptoms can
be shown to have a specific medical cause: epilepsy, a metabolic, or
cardiovascular disorder. Often, even when unable to demonstrate the
presence of diagnostic criteria, the condition is diagnosed as "idio-
pathic epilepsy" and treated with anticonvulsant medication. If the
condition does not reveal underlying organic pathology, it tends to be
regarded as anxiety or hysteria by both non-psychiatrists (family practitioners and neurologists, where most of these patients are seen), and
by psychiatrists and non-psychiatrists alike as a functional disorder
for which there is no specific treatment.

It is particularly when the authority of orthodox medicine is not
demonstrated through production of a specific diagnosis or explanation
that falling-out comes to be viewed by the patient as an "unnatural"
illness with a magical cause. In such instances, any attempts at
treatment, such as tranquilizers or anticonvulsants, will be seen as
inappropriate and irrelevant by the patient, who at this point may feel
the need for a traditional cure. But because of the expense of traditional cures for "unnatural" conditions, because of ambivalent or fear-
ful views of those powers of traditional healers which arise from il-
legitimate sources such as evil spirits, and because of their unintend-
ed but very real "rejection" by the orthodox medical system, these patients may become trapped in continuing illness and increasing debility.

There is no doubt about the reality of falling-out as a culturally
defined (*emic*) condition with specific symptoms. While there may be a
class of individuals with medical or psychiatric diseases who define
their symptoms as falling-out, there is also a group which experiences
falling-out that is not associated with medical disorders. In these
individuals, falling-out appears to be an exclusively dissociative
state which is both psychogenic in origin and characteristic of a
state of altered consciousness. And, like a large and well-recognized
group of "culture-bound" reactive syndromes, it is not classifiable as
conversion hysteria, dissociative hysteria, epilepsy, or a psychotic
reaction. It is, under normal circumstances within its cultural context, an adaptive process designed to handle stress which threatens to
become or is already overwhelming. It appears to be a culturally pat-
terned means of withdrawing from situations that, psychologically,
prove unbearable. However, the potential results of this means of ego-
defense and adaptation may not always be positive, particularly in view
of the life circumstances of poor people and the defensive posture required by the traditional cultural world view. In regressive instances,
falling-out may increase in frequency, duration, and unpredictability.
Individuals then experience increasing debility and possibly even psychogenic death.

Orthodox medical approaches to falling-out do not provide an answer to the problem of conflicting cultural views in health care.
Falling-out of the "unnatural" variety requires spiritual healing at a
minimum, and, when more severe, rootwork. Rootwork is a segmental unit
of a former African religious system (*obeah* is the Bahamian equivalent).

In contrast to such existing, fully organized systems as *vodun* in Haiti, root medicine focuses on malign magical elements and processes which can be used to both send and counteract evil, such as the spiritual forces seen as operating in falling-out of the unnatural variety.

The orthodox medical system has an obligation to treat falling-out, because a restoration of health is one of the functions and purposes of the system. As has been stressed previously, it carries the responsibility for maintaining the health of the nation. From a unicultural view, however, it actually lacks the capacity to treat falling-out that is culturally understood to be unnatural in origin. From the patient's point of view this lack of ability to treat might be considered the equivalent of abandonment and may appear to be a highly arbitrary act of exclusion from appropriate care.

From a transcultural perspective, however, it is conceivable that new referral networks could provide access to traditional healing via the orthodox medical system. By doing so, it is possible to assure the best possible combination of treatments for falling-out of the unnatural type, treatments that give the patient reassurance and meaning by considering his or her health cultural beliefs and practices along with those of standard medical care.

By changing the boundaries of ethical discourse and the parameters within which moral decisions are made, the orthodox health institution exercises legitimate authority that is humane and caring, not arbitrary and dehumanizing. Thus the transcultural perspective allows us to see wherein some of our difficulties lie in providing health care that is equally available and efficacious, regardless of the cultural background of the patient. The transcultural perspective, if utilized within the orthodox health care system, also has the capacity to decrease the dysfunctional aspects of domination that are inherent in a unicultural social institution which is responsible for meeting the health needs of multicultural populations. In ethical terms, the switch from a unicultural to a transcultural perspective means redrawing the limits of our moral community so that both scientifically informed and culturally-informed are included as members participating in ethical discourse related to health and illness. Such a shift in philosophical or value position could go a long way toward returning the orthodox health care system to its position of legitimized dominance and authority because, insofar as cultural factors are concerned, it would no longer be devaluing its ethnic patients or their traditional health cultural systems. This, of course, would free health care providers to act in the best interests of *all* their patients and would function to limit some of the arbitrary uses of power in medical care.

NOTES

1 Hazel H. Weidman, "The Constructive Potential of Alienation: A
   Transcultural Perspective," in *Alienation in Contemporary Society*
   edited by R. S. Bryce-Laporte, and C. S. Thomas, pp. 335-357. (New
   York: Prager Publishers, 1976), citation from p. 343.

2 The concept of *health culture* refers to all of the phenomena associated with the maintenance of well-being and problems of sickness
   with which people cope in traditional ways within their own social
   networks and institutional structures. It is a general term which
   includes both the cognitive and social system aspects of health
   traditions. The *cognitive* dimension involves values and beliefs,
   the blueprints for health action. It requires us to understand
   theories of illness prevention, health maintenance, bodily functioning, disease etiology, diagnosis, treatment, and cure. The *social
   system* dimension refers to the organization of health care or the
   health care delivery system (primarily reparative or therapeutic in
   nature). It requires understanding of the structure and functioning
   of organized sets of health/illness-related roles and behaviors.

3 In the paragraphs to follow, I wish to acknowledge the assistance of
   Mr. Phillip Gordon of the University of Miami School of Medicine.
   Some of the phrasings used in his summaries of my previous publications have been incorporated here. His help in preparing the con-
   densed statement on falling-out (to be introduced below) was particularly valuable.

4 The *emic* view·is that taken from within a particular cultural tradition.

5 The *etic* view is that taken from the vantage point of an observer
   who strives to be objective but who, in fact, brings many of his
   own cultural biases with him. See M. Harris, "History and Significance of the Emic/Etic Distinction," in *Annual Review of Anthropology* edited by B. J. Siegel *et al* 5 (1976), 329-350 (Palo Alto:
   Annual Reviews, Inc.).

6 In French, this would be written, *battement du coeur*; however,
   Haitian Creole transforms the *du* into *de* as we have shown here.

7 Weidman, "The Constructive Potential," p. 346.

8 If the introductory remarks are correct that various evolutionary
   changes have functioned to increase the number of medically "uninformed" persons in contrast to the medically "informed," then processes similar to those described here for ethnic patients and
   orthodox practitioners must be operating also when any medically
   "uninformed" patient interacts with the orthodox, medically "informed" provider of health care.

9 For a full discussion of this syndrome see Hazel H. Weidman, "Falling-Out: A Diagnostic and Treatment Problem viewed from A Transcultural Perspective," *Social Science and Medicine* 13B (1979),
   95-112.

10 Jeffrey C. Rubin and Judy Jones, "Falling-Out: A Clinical Study,"
    Social Science and Medicine 13B (1979), 117-127.

TRADITIONAL CHINESE MEDICINE AND WESTERN MEDICAL PRACTICE:
PERSONAL OBSERVATIONS

ANTHONY K. S. LAM

As a Western-trained medical practitioner I have attempted to understand the philosophy of the causation of disease in Chinese medicine. I have also attempted to apply some traditional Chinese treatments in my practice when I thought they would benefit the patients. Before I discuss my own experiences, I will describe the underlying assumptions and beliefs of Chinese medicine.

The principal relevant theory is the Ying-Yang Theory. Ying has the meaning of negative charge, symbolized by the moon and pertaining to femininity. Yang has the meaning of positive charge, symbolized by the sun, and pertaining to masculinity. So, Ying and Yang have opposite properties. Certain organs in the body belong to Ying and others to Yang. "Solid" organs such as lungs, spleen, heart, and kidneys are Ying organs; "hollow" organs such as intestines, stomach, gall bladder, and urinary bladder are Yang organs. The meridians in acupuncture are also divided into Ying and Yang meridians. When both Ying and Yang are in equilibrium, the person is healthy. When there is a disturbance in the equilibrium, then the person is ill. Groups of symptoms indicate excesses or deficiencies in Ying or in Yang. Strictly speaking, Chinese medicine does not have disease entities such as pneumonia, myocardial infarct, liver cirrhosis, etc. It has sets of symptoms, and when the symptoms disappear, then the illness is "cured." Therefore, its definition of cure is different from ours.

Chinese medicine also emphasizes external factors in the causation of illnesses. They are the wind (風), chills (寒), summer heat (暑), dampness (濕), scorching heat (燥), and fire (火). These terms are even harder for us to understand. The significance of this difficulty is that one must not conclude that some of the Chinese patients, particularly the new immigrants, are irrational when they mention certain peculiar symptoms. Food is also another important factor in causing disease. Some of you in the audience might have been asked by your patients what kinds of food they should avoid. According to the Chinese medical theory, certain foods are to be avoided in every kind of illness.[1]

The diagnostic techniques in traditional Chinese medical practice are based mainly on observation. Traditional physicians look at the colour of the skin, the tongue--its shape, size, teeth indentation, and of course its coating--the sweat, the pulse, the stool, and the urine. Of course, we know and they know, too, that this procedure is not scientific and lacks accuracy. But one has to admire the way they can diagnose diseases from the pulse. They have an elaborate classification in pulse diagnoses. But again it cannot match the modern diagnostic techniques. However, I was quite impressed with one of the doctors in China who diagnosed the illness of my wife when she was coming down with the flu by the palpation of her pulse alone. She had been seeing the doctor for acupuncture treatments for a chronic leg pain. She had no symptoms other than just not feeling quite right that day. The flu diagnosis was merely a coincidental, but accurate finding.

In China today physicians admit the importance of Western medicine. At the same time, they realize that there are valuable contributions from the traditional Chinese medical disciplines. From their formulary, they have medications for such diseases as bronchitis, pyrexia, asthma, gastrointestinal symptoms, and the like. But it was surprising to me that they have medications to dissolve or expel gallstones from the common bile duct. I do not know how effective this treatment would be. Extensive research is being done to uncover the chemical structures of active ingredients of the well-known gin-seng roots, which the Chinese consider the panacea in medicine. They encourage many of their own Western-trained doctors to study traditional Chinese medicine. They even have created a category called "New Medicine" which includes all the new Western diagnostic techniques together with acupuncture.

Chinese physicians also are developing and doing extensive research about acupuncture. They inject a Chinese medication into acupuncture points and along the meridians. They are experimenting with the use of laser beams instead of needles and have been using it in acupuncture anaesthesia. Another interesting technique in acupuncture is the burial of suture materials, mainly cat-gut, in acupuncture points in children with muscle atrophy from polio. They claim that it would increase the muscle mass and strength. Fortunately, this is one technique that would not be of much use in the Western world. But it was sad to see that there are still many small children in China crippled by polio. They claimed that those children are mostly from the rural areas.[2]

I do not see acupuncture anaesthesia to be of wide use in the Western world. The Chinese now admit that when Chairman Mao was still alive, they exaggerated the claims in acupuncture anaesthesia. Even though I have not seen it myself, other Canadian anaesthesiologists have reported that ether anaesthesia is still widely used throughout China, and the Chinese compare ether anaesthesia as the Western method to acupuncture anaesthesia. My impression is that in China today, less than half of the operations are done with acupuncture anaesthesia. The current Western anaesthesia is probably more practical and safer to use than acupuncture in most cases.

However, acupuncture is useful in other ways, and I feel it has a place in Western medicine. It should be used not instead of, but in addition to, other established Western regimens. I have been practicing acupuncture for almost six years, and have achieved great satisfaction in being able to help some of the cases that were literally abandoned by my colleagues. Notice I used the words "some of the cases." Certainly, I have had failures. My statistics will not hold out for one minute in the scientific community, as my results are based solely on the subjective findings of the patients. Hopefully with appropriate funding at a later date, I shall be able to conduct more meaningful experiments. Nonetheless, as far as the patients are concerned, it is only how they feel that counts.

There is nothing mysterious about acupuncture. Just because we do not know how it works, we tend to be skeptical. The magazines and the other news media are partly to blame as they stress the "miracle cure" of acupuncture. For one thing, I explain to all my patients that acupuncture does not cure. It may help to relieve pain either partially or completely, but there is no change in the pathological picture. Stories that one acupuncture treatment completely relieves longstanding pain do occur. I myself have had similar cases, but these are few. The majority of cases require several treatments--the average, between five and ten daily treatments--while some may require twenty to thirty treatments. The effects of acupuncture are not permanent. Periodic treatments are required--sometimes at an interval of several months, and sometimes at an interval of one to two years. This need for further

treatment fits into the present hypotheses in which acupuncture needles
stimulate the release of an intrinsic hormone called "endorphin" which
has analgesic properties.

At present, the legal status of acupuncture in Alberta is confusing. Not too long ago, the College of Physicians and Surgeons of Alberta took a non-medical doctor to court for illegally practicing acupuncture and lost the case. It is my opinion that the practice of acupuncture should be restricted to qualified medical practitioners who
can assess and advise patients if other means of therapy may be more
appropriate, and who can determine whether the patients have been adequately investigated before giving acupuncture treatments. Right now,
medicare does not cover acupuncture treatments. If enough pressure is
put on the politicians, I am sure they will change their minds.

Until more reliable scientific data are available, acupuncture
treatments should be restricted mainly to the relief of pain, as many
of us are now convinced that it is safe and effective. In my practice,
besides using acupuncture for the relief of pain, I have been using it
to help people to stop smoking and the results surprised even me. Our
overall success rate is over 60%, and considering that most patients
require only one treatment, that figure is quite an accomplishment.

In conclusion, I hope I have conveyed to you that if acupuncture
is performed by qualified medical practitioners, it should give us an
additional and an important armamentarium in the treatment of illnesses.

NOTES

1   Wong K. Chimin and Wu Lien-Teh, *History of Chinese Medicine* (Tiet-
    sin, China: Tientsin Press Ltd., 1932).

2   Academy of Traditional Chinese Medicine, *An Outline of Chinese Acu-
    puncture* (Peking: Foreign Languages Press, 1975); Fu Wei-Kang,
    Story of Chinese Acupuncture and Moxibustior (Peking: Foreign
    Languages Press, 1975).

PATIENTS AND PROVIDERS: ALTERNATIVE POWER RELATIONSHIPS
IN A COMMUNITY HEALTH CENTRE

CAROL P. HERBERT

In the past few years, an increasing emphasis has been placed on
consumer involvement and sharing of information and control in health
care. This paper describes the evolution of a community health centre
and power relationships within that facility.

R.E.A.C.H. (Research & Educational Attack on Community Health)
Centre is a community health centre located in Grandview-Woodland, a
multi-ethnic community in east Vancouver, Canada. Opened in 1969
initially as a teaching base for pediatric students when medicare dras-
tically decreased the population of the out-patient department,
R.E.A.C.H. Centre is an innovative teaching, research, and service unit.
R.E.A.C.H. is committed to providing high quality comprehensive continuing medical and dental care with a preventive emphasis, coupled with
teaching of students in the health sciences and research in primary
care. The Centre is funded yearly by the Provincial Ministry of Health
with doctors salaried through the Medical Services Commission and employed by the University of British Columbia Medical School. The current staff consists of five family physicians, two nurse-practitioners,
a clinical pharmacist, a health educator, a nutritionist, a teacher who
co-ordinates a language stimulation program, a clinic co-ordinator and
reception staff; three dentists, and support staff; a clinic administrator, executive secretary, and typist. Additional staff members are
hired for particular programs.

Over the years, R.E.A.C.H. has evolved alternate models of health
care.[1] Before it was fashionable, R.E.A.C.H. explored prevention and
life-style modification, developed nurse-practitioners as care providers, and encouraged self-care and patient involvement in care strategies. We experimented with the health care team concept and, through
trial and error, found practical ways of applying that concept to day-
to-day practice. We created the R.E.A.C.H. Centre Association Board
consisting of a mixture of staff, patients, and community members which
determined policy. We developed community-based projects of diverse
types from a seniors' drop-in pilot project to a day-care Toy Lending

Library. Current community programs include courses in cardio-pulmon-
ary resuscitation, stress management, smoking cessation groups, language stimulation in day-care, a seniors' medication awareness program,
and the toy library.

Our evolution has been determined primarily by the mixture of
health care providers attracted to the Centre. Serendipity, as much as
design, has governed staffing. Staff members have developed programs
and projects according to their interests, with consideration of community need, as assessed by surveys, other area professionals, board
members, and patients. In some measure we have imposed our attitudes
on a community which was not particularly oriented to prevention.

I would like to examine power relationships within the R.E.A.C.H.
Medical Centre from two points of view--the patients and the providers.
The dental practice will not be discussed.

Patients

Initially, our patient population was heavily skewed to young
counter-culture adolescents. In 1970-71, R.E.A.C.H. was the only facility in Vancouver available and responsive to the needs of the transient youth population.[2] In response to high demand (as many as forty
patients an evening in a drop-in clinic), a number of volunteers became involved in delivery of care, including medical, nursing and rehabilitation medicine students, doctors, nurses, lab technicians, and
nutritionists. Initial funding was tenuous, with some staff members on
LIP or OFY funding--federal initiative make-work programs--or research
grants. These early days were critical for the development of an autonomous facility which saw itself as experimental and unbound by models.

Staff was attracted by the opportunity to try new methods and to
deal with different cultures, with the first cross-cultural experience
being the "hippie" culture. A tradition of non-judgmental, respectful
contractual care was begun by necessity. Intrinsic to care provision
at this time was the need to educate the patient. Many of the patients
were non-compliant and rebellious, attitudes characteristic of their
sub-culture. Out of need, we developed strategies for increasing compliance, for accepting our own limitations and patients' limitations,
for education in drug abuse, hepatitis, venereal disease, and birth
control, to name a few areas. We developed alternate strategies for
handling frustration and "sharing care" among non-physician care providers. We attracted physicians who were prepared to share that

control. We developed "adult to adult" transactional methods of com-
municating among the health providers within our facility and with the
patients who attended, rather than the traditional hierarchy of the
hospital with the doctor acting as "parent" to the other staff members.

Acting on us as well was our awareness of and involvement in the
women's self-help movement. We were further affected by the holistic
health movement, by the radical psychiatry movement,[3] by Illich,[4]
Szasz,[5] and others who pointed out the need to share information and
control. We accepted, as a facility, the idea that sharing power with
the patient and among the providers was logical and right, even if
sometimes difficult.

This phase was critical for the development of staff abilities to
deal with our patient mix as it evolved:

(1) Participant-consumers--interested and involved in their own care;
oriented to prevention and lifestyle change; questioning and insistent.
Some of the patients have become involved in the Board. These patients
share Centre philosophy from the outset and are committed to contractual care. They come to R.E.A.C.H. seeking non-authoritarian health
care and expecting to share information and decision-making.

(2) "Victims"--socially displaced or disadvantaged people, including
social agency referrals, alcoholics, addicts, chronic psychiatric patients, and third-generation welfare families--all having in common a
feeling that they are overwhelmed by the social service and medical
system and their own situation to the point where they feel powerless
to change their lives. While such patients are difficult to motivate,
we are experimenting with ways of modifying their sense of themselves
as victims, e.g., by means of stress management groups teaching self-
awareness and self-care strategies.[6]

(3) Traditional users of health care systems--who invest the doctor
with Aesculapian authority[7] but respond to education and information
with behavioral change to varying degrees. This group includes first-
generation ethnic members of our community, in particular, Portuguese,
Italian, and Chinese, and more recently Ugandan and Fijian East Indians. This category also includes some native Indians and some "special
needs" patients, e.g., hearing and sight-impaired. These patients have
in common the problems of:

(a) language and translation,

(b) cultural differences in use of the medical system; in expec-
     tations of the health care providers and in level of compli-
     ance,

(c) suspicion of non-"ethnic" health care workers,

(d) need for extra time for explanation and discussion of their
medical problems,

(e) need for education in the philosophy of patient involvement.

It was our experience with the transient youth of the early seventies that prepared us for dealing with people with multiple problems
and with people from diverse cultures. As the "hippies" were suspicious of the Establishment, so were these subcultures suspicious of the
majority culture. As we wore jeans and involved young volunteers to
make the "hippies" feel at home, so we developed more traditional cos-
tumes and used community volunteers and translators to increase the
comfort of different ethnic groups. As our staff learned the language
and the culture of the "hippies," so we educated ourselves by in-service training on the problem of cultural minorities in the community.
As we adapted to the "hippies'" rebellious avoidance of appointments
and structure, so we developed within the Centre a tradition of flexibility to the ways in which people approach their health care. Over a
longer period, it has become increasingly clear that if we respect the
cultural context of all patients within the Centre, we can assist
people to define their health needs and to use the health care system
more appropriately. Some patients need more time and energy invested
than others to reach that goal.

We have rejected very few patients, absorbing even "hateful" patients more easily than other care settings.[8]

We realized the problems of not having ethnic staff members and
therefore recruited some Italian and Chinese staff. However, it became
apparent that among first-generation Chinese in our community, people
tended to go to Chinese physicians. These patients were not attracted
to our less formal style and preferred more traditional lines of authority. The Italian community is also under-represented in our statistics, though three Italian reception staff members swelled our ros-
ter with family and friends. Again, we were not traditional enough. A
move from our initial makeshift storefront in 1977 to a more profes-
sional-appearing physical plant resulted in increased numbers of Italian patients. As one receptionist put it, "now I'd bring my mother
here"--and she did!

We vacillated between realizing we could never please everybody
and trying to modify our appearance and our behavior to suit tradition-
alists and radicals all at once.

Interestingly, from the outset, we sat in both camps--the radical "hippie clinic" with salaried doctors arousing distrust among community physicians, but at the same time, the University teaching centre with physician staff having medical school and hospital appointments and appearing perfectly "normal" and "ordinary." It was this dual status that allowed us the freedom to develop this unique facility, a part of the University, yet completely autonomous, and also to attract capable committed staff.

I would like to give a few examples of special problems in dealing with multi-ethnic populations and of ways in which we have responded:

(1) A 15-year-old Fijian teenager was found to be twelve weeks pregnant. We advised her that she would have to tell her parents in compliance with the law. She told us she would be beaten by her family-- as indeed she was that same evening. We assisted her in finding temporary housing, but she returned to her family, who sent her to Fiji to have her baby. Afterward, she was ostracized and punished, according to Fijian religious and cultural custom. Because of this patient, we developed in-service teaching around the problems of family breakdown and confusion of sexual mores in the Fijian and East Indian communities and new strategies of early and late intervention.

(2) We recognized that the importance of being "on time" is very much a North American norm, not shared by many other national and cultural groups. We accept the need for someone to see drop-ins every day, particularly among the native Indian population. This provision avoids provider frustration, and ensures care for those patients who never make appointments and for those who come very late or on the wrong day.

(3) For the past two years, we have treated most of the new immigrants to Vancouver who have been found to have parasites on Health Department screening. This treatment requires slow, careful explanation through interpreters and absolute compliance to ensure public protection and completion of immigration formalities. One R.E.A.C.H. physician has assumed this duty because of his interest and his directive skills. Physicians in other standard medical facilities have neither the time nor the inclination for this lengthy intervention.

Providers

Initially, health providers were attracted to R.E.A.C.H. Centre by its innovative approach and by the charisma of its originator and Director from 1969 to 1975, Dr. Roger Tonkin. At that time decision-making was ostensibly at weekly group meetings, but in fact, most important decisions, including all budgeting and most programming initiatives, came from the Director. When he left the Centre, there was a period of turmoil while the whole question of who held the power was re-defined. After initially hiring a second Director, the majority of staff decided that collaborative decision-making was a more appropriate mode. The staff recommended to the Board that the position of Director be replaced by a "co-ordinator" with more restricted power.

From 1976 to 1977, due to budget limitations, the Centre functioned with the clinical pharmacist acting as co-ordinator. During this period, staff and Board re-defined Centre principles and philosophy.

In 1977, a co-ordinator was hired according to a well-defined job description, based on democratic responsibility to staff and Board. During the ensuing three years (1977-1980), the co-ordinator worked on developing a strong community Board. The structure of the Board was modified from a large inactive group to a smaller twelve-person Board with active standing committees. Staff continued to elect voting representatives to the Board (now four of twelve members) and to serve on all committees.

Over the years, we have developed a workable system of whole staff decision-making on matters of policy and programming with feedback to and from the Board. Day-to-day housekeeping and personnel matters are handled by an Executive Committee made up of three elected staff representatives. Some tasks are delegated to specific groups within the staff, e.g., physicians and nurses.

Hiring of staff members is carried out by staff and Board committee selected according to the position to be hired. Staff members are evaluated by written questionnaire and discussion among dental or medical staff at a general meeting at designated intervals (six months and yearly). The budget is constructed by the co-ordinator but approved by both staff and Board. Once the actual budget is received each spring, the staff members determine priorities if cuts need to be made and make recommendations to the Board.

The health professionals have grown to respect each other's skills, to accept the validity of criticism, and to acknowledge the need for review and justification of professional behavior.

At weekly chart review sessions, all providers of care on the medical side are subject to criticism of their management, their prescribing habits, and charting. All members of the team attend these audits. In addition, the clinical pharmacist regularly reviews medication lists on random charts and draws discrepancies to the attention of the prescriber. All charts are reviewed by one of the nurse-practitioners for completeness on the day following a visit.

The physicians are not technically bound by such criticism, as they are employees of the University rather than the R.E.A.C.H. Centre Association, as are all other staff members. However, in practice, physicians have most often voluntarily changed behavior in response to factual criticism by other team members. Occasional problems have arisen when a physician has not modified an attitude or behavior according to group suggestions.

As it may be that perceived physician autonomy has minimized physician turnover compared to other health centres, we have moved cautiously in changing the lines of responsibility.

Within the physician group, decisions are made at monthly meetings and by daily interaction in the office. Each physician carries out designated tasks and responsibilities. No one physician acts as "Medical Director"--the role of director is task-related and changes according to the areas being discussed. For example, one physician acts as liaison with the University, while another physician co-ordinates rounds and meetings. All decisions made by the doctors are subject to discussion and ratification by the staff and Board.

Staff and Board are currently assessing community needs in relation to program development and considering geographic boundaries for new patients because of increasing demand for service. We must determine where energies should be expended--in pilot-program development, continuation of successful programs, direct one-to-one service, and/or research and analysis.

As staff inevitably change, the challenge is to retain flexibility and innovation while becoming increasingly "established" and institutionalized. By remaining a small institution, we hope to maintain our non-hierarchical structure.

Acknowledgements

I wish to acknowledge the secretarial assistance of Lina Fabiano and Joan Chitto in the preparation of this manuscript.

NOTES

1 W. E. Seidelman, B. McMaster and J. Thiel, "A Family-Oriented Approach to Pediatric Care," *Canadian Family Physician* 20 (September, 1974), 62-64; R. S. Tonkin, "The R.E.A.C.H. Centre--Its History and Work (1969-1976) I. Historical Background and Program Description," *Canadian Journal of Public Health* 70 (May/June, 1979), 199-207.

2 C. P. Herbert and J. Thiel, "R.E.A.C.H. Youth Night--The Evolution of an Adolescent Drop-in Program," *Canadian Family Physician* (March, 1975), 79-81.

3 D. Smith and S. David, eds., *Women Look at Psychiatry*, (Vancouver: Press Gang Publishers, 1975).

4 I. Illich, *Medical Nemesis: The Expropriation of Health* (Toronto: McClelland and Stewart, 1975).

5 T. S. Szasz, *The Myth of Mental Illness: Foundations of a Theory of Personal Conduct*, (New York: Dell, 1961).

6 C. P. Herbert and G. M. Gutman, "Practical Group Autogenic Training for Management of Stress-Related Disorders in Family Practice," in *Clinical Hypnosis in Medicine*, (Chicago: Yearbook Publishers, 1980).

7 H. Osmond, "God and the Doctor," *New England Journal of Medicine* 302 10 (March, 1980), 555-558.

8 J. E. Groves, "Taking Care of the Hateful Patient," *New England Journal of Medicine* 298 16 (April, 1978), 883-887.

THE HEALTH CARE TEAM

ACCOUNTABILITY IN THE NURSING PROFESSION

M. JOSEPHINE FLAHERTY

Whenever nurses meet, they express concern about the character of
nursing care that is available and about the quality and quantity of
their own professional practice. As consumers demonstrate increasing
social concern for personal and environmental health, they pose questions about the value of health in relation to other desired goals in
our society. It is crucial for nurses, who face difficult personal and
professional value conflicts, to be able to identify and articulate
thoughtful ethical positions as individual human beings and as professionals. Expansion of the biological sciences has been accompanied by
unprecedented social and cultural changes that have helped to create for
health science professionals new and different dilemmas related to the
use of knowledge and technology to affect human procreation, to modify
behavior, and to influence the course of death. These are bound inex-
tricably to questions about the concepts of health and illness, the
goals of health care, the relationships between patients and those who
care for them, and the efficiency and effectiveness of complex institutions such as the health care system.

Discussion of nursing in Canada today involves a wide variety of
ideas and points of view. The nursing profession exists in response to
a need of society and holds ideals related to man's health throughout
his life span. A concern of the profession is a need to identify and
clarify the unique contribution of nursing to society. Nurses who are
intellectually and practically engaged in the nursing enterprise cannot
help but be involved in attempts to transform nursing knowledge from a
record of unrationalized experiences to a logical organization of relevant phenomena.

Nursing has a long and honored history in Canada. One of the first
health care professionals in this country was Jeanne Mance, Canada's
first nurse, who occupied a position of significance during the early
years of the seventeenth century. At that time, there may have been
only one other health professional, a barber-apothecary, in the country
and no physicians at all. This woman thought and reasoned with accuracy, articulated her beliefs, and had the courage of her convictions.

Like any competent and committed nurse, Jeanne Mance used her energy to
influence all sectors of society--the government, the army, the Roman
Catholic Church, and the people, both Native Canadians and newcomers
from abroad--as she worked to deal with all factors that affected the
health status of the citizens. These factors included their biology,
the environment, their lifestyle, as well as unanticipated events such
as war, accidents, illness, and the health care resources that were
available. Jeanne Mance developed the skills that were necessary for
fulfillment of all aspects of her role as a citizen, a leader, and a
health care worker; these skills even included the ability to use a gun
in the face of war or attack.

Although nursing is discussed a great deal by many people, it is
neither well known nor well understood. It may be that Florence Nightingale was the last person to be sure of what nursing is. In 1860,
Nightingale described nursing as "putting the constitution in such a
state that it will have no disease, or that it can recover from disease."[1] Today, the scope of nursing is regarded as that of health care,
in the broad sense, as opposed to strictly illness care. Its goal as a
field of professional endeavor is to help people attain, retain, and regain health. The phenomena with which nurses are concerned are man's
health-seeking and health-coping behaviors as he strives to attain
health.[2] Nursing in Canada has committed itself to practice according to *nursing* models that lend themselves to change and to adaptation to many venues, as opposed to *medical* or other models. Nurses thus
assess the functional or coping levels of individuals and families in
the light of their biology, their environment, their lifestyle, the
health care system, and the interactions among these; to plan and implement proactive and reactive nursing intervention; and to evaluate the
effectiveness of this activity. Were all nurses able and willing to
identify and assess man's coping behaviors in ways that would facilitate
early and accurate detection of present or potential problems in health
behavior of individuals and groups, the effect of nursing on the health
status of the community could be infinite.

Attempts to define nursing specifically reveal that there is a wide
variety of philosophical, conceptual, and theoretical models under consideration. Each, however, contains certain common threads that include
environmental factors, adaptation factors, and professional interventions. One Canadian nurse has described nursing as a process of nurse-
patient interaction that stems from the assessment of a patient's

needs and levels of functioning and that is designed to optimize the
patient's adaptability through modification and/or reinforcement of the
environment, modification and/or reinforcement of behavior, and biological care and maintenance. This process can be accomplished through
the use of nursing care strategies in appropriate measure.[3]

This type of definition incorporates the notion that nursing practice focuses on the promotion of optimal health for individuals and
families. Health is a manifestation of the competence with which individuals and families function. States of health vary according to the
effectiveness and efficiency with which individuals and families inter-
act with their environments. Hence, health states are measures of functional competence. It follows that if the aim of nursing is to promote
functional competence, nurses in a variety of settings must be expert in
the knowledge, the techniques, and the conceptual and theoretical ra-
tionales that underlie nursing practice.

Nurses of the eighties have declared that they are professional
and that they want to embrace the privileges and responsibilities of
professional status. Probably never before have health care workers,
including nurses, been faced with such complex issues and been called
upon to make such far-reaching decisions. There are certain professional characteristics, possessed by nurses, that have prepared them for
their work.

The first of these is education, both general and specific. General education has provided opportunity for nurses to learn to think and
reason with accuracy, and to develop an appreciation of the world in
which they practice their profession; specific education has provided
a sound theoretical framework for practice. Educational programs have
not been static, but have been modified to meet the needs of students in
the light of the professional demands that will be placed upon them.

A second characteristic of the nursing profession is acceptance of
a code of ethics. Nurses place high value on the worth and dignity of
human beings and that value directs them in their practice. As society
changes and roles are altered, ethical codes may be subject to modification. The basic quality demanded of an ethical professional is integrity, a definition of which was given to me a decade and a half ago by
one of Canada's outstanding medical scientists, who has been demonstrating integrity since before the beginning of this century. To Dr. Peter
Moloney of the Connaught Medical Research Laboratories, acting with integrity means doing what one believes to be right, regardless of the

cost.[4] Belief in something implies that a person has given careful
thought to the information at his or her disposal and has arrived at a
logical conclusion. Beliefs may be modified in the light of new evidence. Competent health professionals, whose philosophies are eclectic
as they borrow from the ancients as well as the moderns for principles
and guidelines, can appreciate the words of Marcus Aurelius who said in
The Meditations:

> A man should always have these two rules in readi-
> ness; the one, to do only whatever the reason of
> the ruling and legislating faculty may suggest for
> the use of men; the other, to change thy opinion,
> if there is anyone at hand who sets thee right and
> moves thee from any opinion. But this change of
> opinion must proceed only from a certain persua-
> sion, as of what is just or of common advantage,
> and the like, not because it appears pleasant or
> brings reputation.[5]

The person with integrity, then, has the courage to change his or her
mind and to admit publicly that he or she was wrong.

A third characteristic of professionals, such as nurses, is dedi-
cation to the ideal of master craftsmanship in their work. The realization of such an ideal involves more than simply being able to do
things well--it requires knowledge and understanding of the principles
on which theory is based as well as the ability to apply these in the
practice of the profession. In *The Metaphysics*, Aristotle said that
"the master craftsmen in every profession are more estimable and know
more and are wiser than the artisans, because they know the reasons of
the things which are done;.... Thus the master craftsmen are superior
in wisdom, not because they can do things, but because they possess a
theory and know the causes."[6] True mastery of a profession is not something that is acquired suddenly. Rather, it is an on-going process that
demands of each professional that he or she strive constantly to add to
personal knowledge, to perfect professional skills, and to enlarge the
body of knowledge for the discipline. The hallmark of a master crafts-
man is an enquiring mind and a commitment to continuous learning.

A fourth characteristic that is part of professionalism is informed
membership and involvement in the organized profession. The member who
is intellectually self-employed thinks and speaks for himself or herself
and acts according to his or her own decisions rather than according to
what someone else has told him or her to do. The member with an enquiring mind knows what is going on in the profession and is involved in the
development of new patterns. He or she will not tolerate the type of
absolutism that is the result of a tired democracy.

The final characteristic, one that subsumes the other four, is accountability, or the taking of responsibility for one's own professional actions. The true professional does not blame others for what has been done or not done in the profession and in the society in which she or he lives. Rather, the professional participates in decision-making and planning and learns to live with the decisions. He or she accepts the fact that failures will be experienced along with successes, but believes that if he or she acts responsibly, the successes will outnumber by far the failures. The professional strives constantly to practice in a diligent, reasonable, and justifiable manner, to document his or her reasoning, and to display a willingness to subject it to the scrutiny of peers. Thus health professionals, who no longer feel obliged to carry the burden of omniscience, develop and apply strategies to deal with almost instant obsolescence of knowledge and professional practice and achieve "Maturity: that means among other things--not to hide one's strength out of fear and, consequently, live below one's best."[7] An accountable nurse's "best" performance involves exercise of professional practice, through application of the nursing process, at the highest level at which the nurse is capable. The nursing process, for which Canadian nurses are responsible, is composed of at least four dimensions: planning, implementation, evaluation, and research. Careful attention must be given to these, each of which is subject to being affected markedly by the far-reaching scientific and technological advances of our age and by actual and hoped-for changes in the delivery of health care.

Planning involves the recognition of real or potential problems or needs of patients and the identification of strategies for coping with these. Planning may be narrowed to one or more individuals or broadened to a department, an institution, or a community. Implementation involves decisive action towards a defined goal. It can become routinized, cold, almost mechanical, but it has the potential to be the most creative, communicative, and satisfying component of the nursing role. It is the "art of nursing." Evaluation is the process of determining the significance or worth of nursing action by careful appraisal and study. It should involve also the determination of appropriateness. It takes place concurrently with and retrospectively to implementation, as well as prior to new planning. One of the marks of a profession is that it monitors its own practitioners; thus, accountable nurses must be prepared for peer review as well as self-evaluation. Research involves disciplined study of the effects of nursing actions that will lead to

the development of non-arbitrary standards for nursing practice, standards that are developed by specialists in nursing rather than by administrative or organizational tradition or convenience.

This professional scope of nursing embraces three complementary
aspects: The first is the *independent* function, in which the nurse
makes judgments that are based on education and experience and that depend on sound theoretical knowledge. The second is the *dependent* function, in which the nurse acts according to the directions of physicians
or other health professionals and according to policies of health care
agencies. The nurse in Canada is obliged by ethics and by law to question those directions and policies about which he or she has concern.
The third is the collaborative or *interdependent* function, in which the
nurse works with patients, families, and other members of the health
care team in the effort to meet patients' needs. This requires mutual
respect and co-operation among health care workers.

According to provincial laws, to ethical codes, and to standards
of professional practice, nurses in Canada are significantly independent
professional practitioners of health care who are *accountable for* their
behavior, rather than *accountable to* someone in a hierarchy. Under
these provisions, every registered nurse must exercise judgment in accepting responsibility and is accountable for his or her own actions.
The acts of registered nurses require substantial knowledge, skills, and
judgment and are performed either independently or in co-operation with
other members of the health care team.

In some jurisdictions, recognition of the autonomy of the nursing
profession and of its responsibility for regulation of itself as a profession may be explicit in the statutes, whereas in others, this acknowledgment is implicit. There is general agreement, however, that nursing
is a distinct profession that involves the three dimensions of the nursing function.

The ethical implication of this statutory and professional
context for nurses, whether they are engaged in nursing practice,
nursing education, nursing administration, nursing research, or
consultation, is that they are accountable for professional behavior
that involves application of the nursing process and co-operation with
appropriate others, within current legislation affecting the practice of
nursing, according to the profession's codes of ethics and of practice
and within the context of the policies and practices of the employing
institution. This requires nurses, along with other professionals, to

practice with competence and to exercise judgment in the preservation of
the safety, dignity, and autonomy of patients. While few people would
neglect safety and dignity, nurses, like many other professionals who
establish practices modelled on the system under which they were trained, must guard against being tempted to slip into an Aesculapian model
in which goals are defined *for* patients rather than *with* them. Current
conceptual models of nursing practice do not direct nurses to sustain
hope in health care recipients by promises of survival or cure of
disease (that patients often know is not possible); rather, these models
direct nurses to sustain hope by keeping patients as much in command of
themselves, their symptoms, and their situations as possible and thus
preserving the autonomy of patients. Autonomy calls for a degree of
independence or freedom or choice for the individual; it requires for
that person knowledge, ability to reason, and ability to act in a way
that is true to his or her nature. No one is truly autonomous; everyone
needs and depends somewhat on others to authenticate his or her acts, to
provide knowledge, to assist with thinking, and to facilitate choices.
In health care, the relationship between the professional and the patient is a medium by which autonomy can be enhanced. Professionals
succeed in the preservation of autonomy when those patients requiring
continuing care are able to function with the least possible interference from their disease or their therapeutic regime.[9]

In the eighties, perhaps more than ever before, ethical nurses will
have to go beyond direct patient care to consider and act upon factors
associated with the nature and shape of the health care system, the
responsibilities and practices of various members of the health care
team, and the changing roles of consumers in the maintenance of their
own health. Nursing will continue to promote the adaptation of patients
in situations where changes in health status (including but not restricted to illness) place new demands on those patients.

Nurses are conscious that whatever they observe about their patients, and how the patients perceive what is happening to them, will be
influenced by the setting in which it occurs and by the forces, obvious
and subtle, that the setting contains. The education and experience of
nurses have prepared them to subject all nursing phenomena to the analytic scrutiny that is part of the nursing process: nursing professionals
look at individual trees as well as the woods. This component of excellent nursing practice goes beyond the mere counting, reducing to numerical scores, and checking off on lists of the results of observation

(that Florence Nightingale identified as a nurse's most necessary skill), and implies a subjective determination. Rather than being whimsical or unreasoned, however, such a determination involves the combination of all parts into a meaningful whole in which theoretically and technically skilled and personally and socially perceptive health care practitioners engage as they make clinical judgments.

As they do this, nurses will examine the results of biological, medical, technical, and social advances that would have been inconceivable to their predecessors. This examination may shake, if not shatter completely, certain personal and professional beliefs that most of them value highly, such as convictions about the dignity of human life, the uniqueness of each human being, and the freedom of every individual to control his or her life and lifestyle. As members of society and as practitioners, nurses may have to re-think and re-define their purposes, their nature, and their value systems. To do this, they will require personal philosophies that are meaningful to them, explicit definitions of their ethical beliefs, identification of their own personal--professional conflicts, and acknowledgment of the extent to which they are imposing these on others and to which these conflicts affect the health care being provided.

Through demonstrated and recognized competence and productivity in intellectual arenas and through the pursuit of excellence in nursing practice, nurses in this country have earned membership in the scientific community. They are driven to find new means to explore what is not yet known in nursing and to develop and test new strategies and novel approaches to health care problems. Nurses have knowledge and experience that suggest directions for care.

The National Research Council of the United States has noted that because of their "tradition, natural inclination, and previous training. . .nurses view health problems differently and direct the results of their research to quite different audiences than other biomedical and behavioral scientists."[10]

Nurses at all levels recognize that the direction of scientific discovery and its application to mankind are not out of their hands. They have personal, professional, and legal responsibilities to ask probing questions about scientific and technical research and its application (or lack of it) in practice. Each health professional and each patient must be given the right, without censure or humiliation, to hear a drumbeat different from that of others. Nursing practice

must be directed by a genuine concern for a patient's own worth, for
him or her as a person, regardless of that patient's social values and
capacity for achievement. This may appear to be a tall order but it is
a professional imperative for nurses who allege that their hallmark is
the caring quality of their behavior.

It is because of the increasing number of "thinking doers" in
nursing that the spirit of enquiry is spreading up and down the nursing
ranks and is not reserved for a nursing elite. The challenge to nurse
teachers is to demonstrate to students, and educate them in, the practice of critical thought that, if real, is on-going and not merely epi-
sodic. The challenge to nurse-managers is to create environments in
which nurses in all types of positions can think critically with im-
punity and hence be able to make the "imaginative leap that transforms
an undifferentiated given into a pattern of reason."[11] The challenge
to the researcher is to see the implications for nursing practice of
the basic observations of nurses and to investigate the relevant questions.

All responsible members of the profession, who work in various
settings in nursing, will be involved constantly in critical appraisal
of what they are doing. This includes definition of objectives, speci-
fication of the conditions under which these objectives can be met,
followed by location, and if necessary, creation of these conditions,
the taking of nursing actions in appropriate measure to meet the objectives, rigorous evaluation of the results of the actions, and implementation of modifications in nursing strategies where indicated.

Obsolescence of professional nursing practice is almost as trouble-
some a problem today as is the obsolescence of machines. Since nurses,
like other professionals, must use training and experience received in
the past to meet present and future practice needs, they strive constantly to remain in touch with the worlds of relevant nursing theory
and practice. There is a need today, perhaps to a greater extent than
ever before, for nurses to "think out loud" in the presence of their
peers in order to expose their ideas, at all stages of development, to
the scrutiny and critical thought of their fellows.

Nurses were reminded by Romanell that the guiding principle for
ethical nursing behavior is epitomized in the words of Socrates in
Plato's *Apology*: "The unexamined life is not worth living."[12] The examined life is lived today by those nurses who are willing to question
the prevailing customs and taboos of the situations in which they find

themselves, including their own behavior, to identify whether what they see is consonant with the standards of practice for which they stand accountable.

This challenges the responsible nurse to subject established methods, policies, and institutions, including codes of ethics and tried and proven methods of acting, to constructive criticism in an effort to determine the need to transform the old order into a new and better one. This will not provide clear-cut mechanisms for the solution of all dilemmas of nursing practice. However, it can stimulate the nursing practitioner to strive for excellence in his or her own practice, to apply traditional ethical concepts that are adaptable to the culture or cultures in which he or she works and thus to make appropriate decisions when faced with professional and ethical dilemmas.

NOTES

1 Florence Nightingale, *Notes on Nursing: What it is and what it is not* (New York: Dover Publications, 1969), p. 4.

2 Rozella Schlotfeldt, "This I Believe. . .Nursing is Health Care," *Nursing Outlook*, 20, 4, (April, 1972), 245.

3 Adaptation of definition after personal communication with Professor Marian McGee, Faculty of Nursing, University of Western Ontario, London, 1975.

4 Personal communication with Dr. Peter Moloney, Senior Scientist, Connaught Medical Research Laboratories, Toronto, 1962.

5 Marcus Aurelius, *The Meditations*, trans. George Long, IV, 12 (Garden City, New York: Doubleday, 1960), p. 37.

6 Aristotle, *The Metaphysics Book I*, trans. Hugh Tredennick, 1, 11-12 (London: Heinemann, 1933), p. 7.

7 Dag Hammarskjold, *Markings* (London: Faber and Faber, 1966), p. 87.

8 Eric J. Cassell, "Autonomy and Ethics in Action," *New England Journal of Medicine*, 297 (1977), 333-334.

9 *Ibid.*

10 *Personnel Needs and Training for Biomedical and Behavioral Research: The 1977 Report of the Committee on the Study of National Needs for Biomedical and Behavioral Research Personnel.* Commission on Human Resources, National Research Council, Vol. I. (Washington, D.C.: National Academy of Sciences, 1977), 152.

11 James Dickoff, Patricia James and Joyce Semradek, "8-4 Research. Part I: A Stance for Nursing Research--Tenacity or Inquiry," *Nursing Research*, 24 2 (March-April, 1975), 85.

12 Patrick Romanell, "Ethics, Moral Conflicts and Choice," *American Journal of Nursing*, 17, 5 (May, 1977), 850.

A PROLEGOMENON TO THE ALLOCATION OF RESPONSIBILITY IN HIERARCHICAL ORGANIZATIONS: NURSES AND PHYSICIANS*

BENJAMIN FREEDMAN

I

Introduction

After entry into a hospital, a patient certainly has much more contact with nurses than with physicians; and a physician, for that matter, is likely to have much more to do with nurses than with patients. Nurses are the missing middle term in discussions of medical ethics, which tend to concentrate upon physician-patient interactions, to the relative exclusion of patient-nurse or nurse-physician relationships. The significance of these latter relationships for ethical understanding cannot be denied, particularly for the analysis of physicians and authority, yet they suffer from a paucity of ethical discussion.

This gap in the literature can be understood in the light of another factor. The ethical issues surrounding nursing practice fall under the topic of the allocation of responsibility in hierarchical organizations. Conceptually, understanding the health-care team is analogous to understanding corporations or, at the extreme end of the scale, the military.

Ethical theorists are most comfortable with very simple models of responsibility: primarily, with what we might call monadic functions. These apply when we want to know whether an individual who has performed an action is responsible for that action. This simple theoretical paradigm is concerned with individuals who are acting on their own: ethical entrepreneurs.

This model is not adequate to cover individuals who are acting in a corporate capacity (in the broad sense). Possibly because of the difficulties encountered in describing monadic responsibility, models for more complicated situations have scarcely been attempted. Yet lacking such models, it is futile to discuss the ethics of corporate actors: nurses, executives, soldiers. And so these fields have lain fallow.

*A revised version of this paper has appeared in the *Legal-Medical Quarterly*, 4 (Spring, 1981), 35-43.

I am interested in presenting many questions and some preliminary
conclusions on the allocation of responsibility in hierarchical organizations. My particular concern is to describe these questions in their
application to the case of nurses. As already indicated, though, the
topic is far broader. The historical trend has been to expand the number of choices for action which arise in organizational settings, at the
expense of those ethical choices which we face in our private capacities. These questions, unbeknownst to academics, are becoming the norm.
They need to become the core of ethical inquiry.

II

Preliminaries

What do we mean when we speak of the allocation of responsibility?
What are we distributing when we distribute responsibility?

There are at least two senses which are relevant here. One common
sense of responsibility is liability or blame. When something goes
awry, and we know who is responsible for it, then we know who ought to
pay--whether payments be made in dollars, in punishments, or in bearing
moral guilt.

But responsibility as liability assumes that something goes wrong,
and although writers tend to deal with that case, it is in a way a
secondary concern. We should first of all be clear about what things
look like when they go right. "Initial responsibility" concerns those
chores and duties which are assumed by an individual upon joining an
organization. There is no simple logical maneuver which enables us to
move from initial responsibility to liability (or blame) responsibility,
or vice versa. I will deal with these two forms of responsibility
separately. There are still other senses of responsibility--e.g., caus-
al responsibility.[1] I am not interested in these other senses in themselves, but rather in the contribution they can make to elucidation of
the two forms of responsibility already introduced.

Another relevant distinction is that between legal and moral responsibility. Inasmuch as society has tried to forge a morally acceptable system of law, a considerable overlap between the two is to be
expected. They are, however, separate topics, and I am concerned with
moral responsibility, although the law may yield some useful guidance
for this topic.

By a "hierarchical organization" I mean nothing more than an employing institution, in which some employees stand to others as superior
to subordinate. Communes are one type of organization which is excluded. Certainly many questions on the definition and description of
hierarchical organizations suggest themselves, but in this paper I will
take the concept as a given.

III

Excuses: Orders From Above

The responsibility of one committing an immoral act under a superior's orders is the richest source on this topic in the literature. The
claim has been advanced--in the Eichmann case, for example, and in the
My Lai investigations--that an actor within a hierarchical organization
is not subject to the same principles of blame as is one who acts independently. This is, then, a question of liability responsibility: Do
superior orders exculpate? It is, of course, a question which a nurse
often confronts. Should she follow a physician's orders if they appear
immoral?--e.g., an order to lie to a cancer patient about diagnosis and
prognosis. If apparently immoral orders have been obeyed, is the nurse
free of blame?

Most systems of law have confronted this problem, without however
affording a great deal of clarification. One interesting instance is
that of *halakha*, Jewish law. A well-entrenched principle in Jewish law
has it that blame cannot be transmitted through an intermediary.[2] That
is to say, if one orders you, or engages you, to commit an unlawful act,
no agency has been established. The one performing the transgression
cannot impute his act to another. The rationale of this principle is
given in the form of a rhetorical question: The words of the master and
the words of the student: to whose words does one listen?

However, there are established exceptions to this general principle. There is Biblical evidence that agency for a transgression is
established if the principal is the king.[3] Other exceptions are discussed in the Talmud.[4]

The common law is even more murky on this question. It upholds a
general principle, which we might term the opacity of responsibility, a
principle which is widely held among writers in ethics as well. The
principle has it that the chain of responsibility is broken by the action of an agent, so that it is in general the last person, the one who
consummates the harm, who bears liability responsibility.

Yet in spite of this principle, in both tortious and criminal liability we can find the opposed idea of "inducing" action, in which case
the liability is imputed not to the actor but to the one who "caused"
him to act.[5] In an instance in which one is commanded to act by another
in a position of authority, the law speaks of "coercion." So, for example, the captain of a vessel who ordered an infirm sailor to go aloft
was held guilty of manslaughter when the seaman fell to his death.[6]

It is surely not the mere fact that you have been ordered to act
by a superior which serves to exculpate. Moral responsibility cannot
be subject to morally irrelevant factors, such as the job which is held.
How is it that even a *prima facie* case for an excuse can be generated
out of this situation?

There are a number of factors, which fall under three classifica-
tions, which can be put forth as either mitigating (reducing blame) or
exculpating (removing blame). The first classification concerns coercing and enticing factors; the second, factors which create a justified
reliance on the judgment of a superior; the third, factors which serve
to mask the nature of the moral choice faced.

A. Coercing and Enticing Factors

The factors in this classification are predicated upon the greater
power of the superior to affect your personal situation, for good or
ill. With some violence to ordinary language, we could speak of one
being "coerced" into doing wrong when he is threatened with some substantial harm if he does not obey the command; and of one being "enticed" into wrong if he faces some substantial benefit for compliance.

Of course, both of these factors may be present in a particular
case. A nurse is ordered to falsify a patient's chart, to cover up a
physician's negligence. She may be coerced into this, if failing the
emendation, she will lose her job; she is enticed if, subsequent to
the emendation, she will be recommended for promotion; if both sets of
consequences are promised, she is both coerced and enticed.

Can these factors mitigate blame? It would seem that they can. In
inquiring into the seriousness of a wrong, we inquire into the motives
of the actor; and surely the motives of the nurse here--to hold onto her
job--are understandable, if self-serving. They are surely better than
the physician's motives: he faces his dismal choice by his own fault,
but she has been forced into the choice she faces.

Might these factors serve to exculpate? This is a more difficult
question. One is inclined to appeal to a sliding scale, which varies
across two vectors: the seriousness of the harm committed, and the
seriousness of the consequence faced. Perhaps there is exculpation if
one is faced with loss of one's livelihood consequent upon refusal to
commit a peccadillo. The question is this: Can we expect a sincere,
well-intentioned person to resist the order?

In those instances of very serious personal consequences and very
minor immorality, it would seem to me that exculpation is possible. We
must remember that we are here dealing with the theory of blaming, not
ideal ethical theory. Surely one who resists the order in these situations has done a better thing than one who avails himself of the excuse; the former has in fact done something praiseworthy. Yet in calling this action praiseworthy, we indicate its supererogatory nature,
the fact that it goes beyond duty. One has not done anything wrong in
not performing an act of supererogation (though one has failed to do
something right); and so, it appears that *following* orders in the indicated circumstances is excusable.

But there is no obvious criterion of equality between consequence
and wrong which may be adopted. We tend to blame Eichmann, surely, even
though the coercion--possible execution--was extreme. Nor do I believe
there would be exculpation if one faces death for not killing another.[7]

Another source of unclarity here is the question of how seriously
ought we to take enticements, as opposed to coercion. Can even the enticement of a great reward exculpate the performance of even a minor
transgression? I am inclined to think not. Even if enticements have no
moral competence to impute one's action to another, we still are left
with a problem, for it is often unclear whether a proffered consequence
should be seen as a threat or benefit. Imagine that you are unemployed,
and are offered a job for committing this wrong: is the job an unal-
loyed benefit, or a veiled threat ("Do this or I won't hire you.")?
Does it make a difference whether or not the job is one for which you
are qualified? Is it relevant fact that you had earlier been promised
the job? I have elsewhere[8] discussed these questions, and have suggested that if the "benefit" is something to which you are morally entitled, it should be seen as a veiled threat: Do this immoral act, or
remain where you are--while "where you are" is in a situation which is
itself morally unjustified. Nevertheless, clearly these questions require further discussion.

B. Factors Creating A Justified Reliance

One of the facets of organizations which complicates our topic
stems from the form of authority which a superior has over another. For
it is authority which is often in question, not bare power. Superiors
are obeyed not only out of fear, but out of respect.

The second group of factors, then, which represent possibilities
for excuse in obeying orders are factors which caused the subordinate
to rely upon the judgment of the one giving the order. There are numerous permutations possible here. He may have dealt with the superior
over a long period of time, and found that his judgment is trustworthy;
further, he may have questioned some of the superior's judgments in the
past, only to find out later that the superior was right. Or, one may
have had no dealings with this individual in the past, but the position
occupied by the superior and the general respect which he has garnered
may justify one in relying upon his judgment. Both of these factors are
often present for nurses: the position which the physician occupies in
the medical setting and in the society at large is one of respect and
authority.

Surely there are instances in which we are justified in relying upon another's moral judgment, or even in substituting another's judgment
for one's own. But just as surely, there are limits to how far this can
be taken.

One such limit has been pointed to by Robert Veatch, in his coining
of the phrase, "the generalization of expertise."[9] The physician's expertise in questions of medicine does not necessarily carry over to confer upon him an expertise in questions of medical ethics. A nurse's
proper attitude towards a doctor is not one of generalized awe, and care
must be taken that acceptance of an authority's judgment on matters falling within his competence does not slide over to a general acceptance of
his judgment. No excuse lies when accepting a superior's judgment in
his areas of incompetence, or unproven competence.

(Yet the application of these ideas to concrete situations is not
simple, for questions of medical ethics have an important empirical component, and in that area the physician's competence may well be present.
In telling the nurse to give a false prognosis to this patient, the
physician likely believes that telling the patient the truth will harm
him in some way. A nurse's doubt about carrying out this order *might*
be predicated upon a different empirical belief than that held by the

doctor; and the nurse might be justified in substituting his estimation
of the chances for harm for her own.)

Another limit to the substitution of judgment would occur when the
question at hand is clearly moral in nature, and one on which the nurse
has strongly-held ethical views which are in clear conflict with those
of the doctor. If you are commanded to perform an act which seems to
you clearly immoral--e.g., to falsify a patient's chart so that the
physician's malpractice will remain concealed--then any past presumption
that the physician's moral judgment is trustworthy has been defeated.
Your present, as well as your past, experiences with an individual enter
into a justified appraisal of character. In instances in which you are
not justified in thinking someone morally trustworthy, you are not excused in adhering to that individual's moral judgment.

This exception, together with the earlier one, suggest that one may
rely upon another's judgment with regard to information, or concrete
moral questions which mix issues of fact and principle, but never upon
another's judgment on pure questions of moral principle. If so, this is
a recent development. Historically, people have often substituted
another's moral conscience for their own. I am not sure whether contemporary moral attitudes in this regard are a positive or negative development. Perhaps each opposed attitude is proper given differing historical contexts.

In saying that justified reliance is possible upon information,
but not upon moral principles, an interesting analogy suggests itself.
In Roman law, as in our legal system today, ignorance of the law does
not excuse, while ignorance of fact does excuse.

C. Masking Factors

The nature of institutions is such that not merely power, but information as well, is allocated according to one's position in the
hierarchy. This allocation may be predicated upon many factors: it
might be that only at certain levels are the individuals sufficiently
trained to evaluate or comprehend information; it might be that for institutional reasons, which may be benign or malignant, it is desired
that there be a restriction in informational flow.

At times, then, the true nature of the moral choice is one which
is only available to superiors, and so no blame could be attached to
one who is following orders. For example, the engineer in charge of a
nuclear station who orders a technician to release some radioactive

gases into the atmosphere has placed the technician in this sort of
position. The technician is, perhaps, unable to make an evaluation of
safe levels of radiation release; moreover, he may be incompetent to
judge the harmful consequences which would ensue from failing to release
the radiation as ordered. One of the most firmly established conclusions in ethical inquiry has it that blame must be judged from the point
of view of the actor in question, with due regard to his factual beliefs
and the reasonableness of his holding them.

The case of factors which mask the nature of the moral choice
faced is the extreme case of factors which create a justified reliance
upon the superior's judgment. In justified reliance, one suspends one's
judgment concerning certain facets of action in favor of another's beliefs; in masking factors, one has no choice but to rely upon the
other's judgment. In fact, if the nature of the choice has been sufficiently masked, one is not even aware of any significant moral dimension
to the choice faced. The only way to blame one who acted in a masked
situation is by showing that his blindness was willful, was his own
fault, was in itself culpable in some way; and then the guilt attaches
not to the action, but to dereliction in a different area: in not
learning all that should have been learned.

In traditional accounts of liability responsibility--the theory of
blaming--one is held to account if: the act performed is harmful, or
otherwise morally objectionable, as an act; if it was done willfully,
voluntarily; and if it was done with knowledge that it is a wrongful
act. My discussion has taken for granted that the act in question is
wrongful; otherwise, no excuse would be necessary. Given the wrongfulness of the act, factors of coercion and enticement may more or less
impair the free action of the will, and so may either exculpate or mitigate blame in varying degrees. The masking factors, and the factors
creating a justified reliance upon another's judgment, relate to the informational requirement of blame; the first refers to easily-described
knowledge which only the superior possesses, and the second to inchoate
knowledge imputed by the inferior to the superior.

It is possible that this requirement is an all-or-nothing affair,
and so these factors would either be void or would exculpate. The only
way in which they might appear to be mitigating factors would be by
judging the situation faced by the subject to be other than the situation which we felt to be in question. This would not be a true mitiga-
tion: instead of excusing in part one's action, it explains that a

different, blameable, action is in question. (There was no attempted murder; it was really an aggravated assault.) Whether this is true or not, though, it would seem that insofar as blaming relates to wrongfulness, will, and information, other excusing factors arising from the nature of action in hierarchical organizations could be subsumed under one of the categories introduced here.

One final word about the topic. A possible parallelism which ought to be explored is that between blame and praise. If one lays oneself open to blame in executing the immoral order of a superior, does one become a subject of praise in performing a laudatory action under orders? And, are the excusing conditions for blame also "excusing" conditions for praise? Certainly this would be the case with regard to the informationally-connected factors (justified reliance and masking factors), for in those instances your action is a morally and conceptually thin one, in its having been performed without adequate knowledge of the action's ramifications. Would this also be the case with regard to coercing and enticing factors? It might be particularly rewarding to explore this possible parallel because praise is so less emotionally loaded a topic than is blame.

IV

Initial Responsibility

Liability responsibility represents responsibility's pathology, while initial responsibility reveals the structure of a well-run system. Initial responsibility has to do, as remarked earlier, with the allocation of chores and duties in an organization. This, as any task, can be done well or foolishly; if done well, it eliminates many problems which arise at the level of pathology.

Two separate questions relate to initial responsibility. The first has to do with how responsibility can be well allocated at the origin of an organization. The second concerns the discernment and adjustment of initial responsibility in already extant institutions. That there are two questions here is the result of an ambiguity in the phrase "initial responsibility," in which "initial" might apply to the beginning of the institution, or to the beginning terms of employment.

Let us start with the first question. Starting with a clean slate, how ought organizational charts be formulated so as to properly allocate responsibility?

Factors from the previous section are certainly of relevance. In assigning a role, one wishes to ensure that the conditions of employment (e.g., educational attainment and previous work experience) stand in a rational relationship to the power which will be wielded and the informational requirements which will need assimilation. Rationality forbids underqualification (though it may permit overqualification).

Along a different dimension, a relevant factor might be called sleeping in the bed which you have prepared. For reasons of prudence--to help ensure proper fulfillment of the assigned responsibilities--it is desirable that the one who is required to clear up the messes be the one who has created them.

If these factors are indeed relevant (they are certainly not exhaustive) one is equipped to deal with the second question; in particular, with the criticism of the way in which responsibility is currently allocated.

Take the current relative status of physicians and nurses. To an outsider, it seems that this relationship is badly distorted due to the presence of a (possibly unconscious) model. The model I have in mind is that of master and servant. In it, the essential responsibility for successfully managing the patient is in the hands of the doctor. The nurse's role is almost exclusively that of conscientiously carrying out the doctor's instructions. This model might be a historical carry-over from a time in which the nurse was, typically, the doctor's employee, just as the doctor's secretary was his employee. Under this model, all of a nurse's professional responsibilities are duties of obedience. In failing to carry out an order, she is in intrinsic breach of her duty to carry out the terms of her employment, a duty with some moral weight. This is not to say that under this model it is never right for a nurse to disobey, for one is often obliged to breach one moral duty in adherence to a more important one. It does mean, however, that each time a nurse is confronted with an immoral order she is faced with a moral dilemma.

It is a moot question whether this model was ever accurate, but it is surely not accurate today. Nursing is an autonomous discipline, with its own values, goals, and educational process. It must be defined in its own terms, and not merely as a profession adjunctive to physicians. Since that is so, there must, logically, be areas of initial responsibility which should be granted to nurses. Simply put, the nurse is often the best-trained for the job. A rational scheme of initial allocation will recognize this.

Which jobs the nurse is best qualified to perform is an empirical
question. Likely candidates are those chores which require empathy,
since the nurse's involvement with a patient is likely to be more extensive, and hence better informed, than the physician. (To some extent,
this claim is not today as true as it ought to be. Because of our mis-
apprehension that the doctor should be the primary bearer of initial responsibility, he is allocated tasks such as talking extensively with the
patient and the patient's family, which provide him with opportunities
for insight which are currently denied to the nurse.) I think a plausible, but controversial, suggestion to offer at this point is this: the
nurse ought to bear primary initial responsibility for communication, at
least in the case of the long-term, chronically hospitalized patient.
My hesitation over extending this to the entire patient population has
to do with the possibility that in short-term encounters communication
is appropriately confined to narrow, technical medical matters, and on
these matters the physician is more likely to be expert.

This proviso, though, is a matter to be determined by factual investigation. So is the question of what other tasks are more appropriately carried out by nurses than by physicians.

Among the problems which this suggestion brings to mind is that of
possible supersessionary power on the part of superiors in general; in
our case, on the part of physicians. Given that the nurse is given
primary initial responsibility for communication, we have not theoretically blocked off the possibility that the doctor ought to possess veto
power over the exercise of this power. Whether or not this power ought
to be granted is elucidated by getting clear about the possibilities for
overlap. If, for example, the physician's initial responsibility includes the medical management of the patient, and if communication can
seriously impact upon this (as of course it can), then veto power would
be in order. This veto would not return things to the unsatisfactory
status quo ante; for a veto would have to be seen in the nature of an exception under this proposed model. In general, the *presence* of supersessionary power indicates a superior-subordinate relationship, not the
exercise of this power.

V

Full Compliance and Partial Compliance

Sometimes theories are designed upon the notion that all of their strictures will be adhered to; these are called full compliance theories. At other times, factors are introduced into the theory to take account of possible violations; these are partial compliance theories.

A full description of the theory of the allocation of responsibility in hierarchical organizations needs to perform both tasks. The section on initial responsibility can be seen as addressing itself to full compliance; the section on excuses is, of course, appropriate to a partial compliance theory.

A classical issue of partial compliance theories which needs exploration is whistle-blowing. In the event that you know of an individual who has neglected his duty, what ought you to do? We are concerned with derelictions of moral duty, which may or may not involve negligent job performance.

Conceptually, whistle-blowing is an issue distinct from that of the excuse from superior orders. Practically speaking, however, the two issues raise much the same questions.

An important clue to this practical point is found in the fact that we think of the problems in an inferior blowing the whistle on a superior, not vice versa. Given that we are interested in moral dereliction of duty, why should this be so? A job does not, after all, confer a privileged moral status.

The answer must be that there is a clear moral responsibility to blow the whistle. Because of this clear responsibility, it seems to us obvious that a superior ought not hesitate in calling to task his subordinate. The only reason why there is any moral question about whistle-blowing at all is that, when a subordinate might call to account his superior, he has available all of the excuses which were earlier noted in reference to excuses stemming from orders from above: consequent upon the structure of the organization are factors which coerce, entice, create a justified reliance, or mask the true nature of the moral situation.

Whistle-blowing will yield to much the same tactics as were earlier employed. Certain modifications must of course be made. For example, in whistle-blowing one's estimation of the personal consequences is less reliable than in superior orders: first, because whistle-blowing does

not involve a clear breach of the chain of command; second, because the
feared consequences of whistle-blowing are likely to emanate from a number of people--other superiors, and even one's peers--in contrast to a
violation of orders, when the primary object of fear is the superior.
As another example, we might note that the excuse from justified reliance becomes relatively more important for whistle-blowers than for
those following superior orders. Those who argue against whistle-blowing by appeal to the language of loyalty to and trust in one's superiors
are in fact appealing to those factors which create justified reliance.
But these points represent empirical adjustments, rather than disparate
principles.

Another topic needing further discussion has to do with the relationship between initial responsibility and blame (liability) responsibility. The practical question is whether one's initial responsibilities impact upon the excuses which are traditional in hierarchic organizations.

Again, in the spirit of tentative conclusions, I would suggest that
initial responsibility serves as an aggravating factor in blame, and
tends to nullify the effect of excusing conditions. Should a nurse be
ordered by a physician to communicate immorally to a patient (on the
earlier assumption that communication is one of her initial responsibilities), the order ought to be resisted. Since she has been given initial responsibility because of the presumption that she is the most
competent individual on these matters, the factors which appeal to the
subordinate's disadvantaged information position (justified reliance and
masking) are unavailable to excuse. Coercing and enticing factors are
also weaker, because the harmful consequences attach more intimately to
the nurse in that they are violations of her professional *raison
d'être*.[10]

The same comments are apposite to issues of whistle-blowing. Your
obligation to call a superior to task is clearly greater when he has
appropriated one of your tasks and been derelict in this performance
than when he has wrongly carried out a task of his own.

One reason for the relationship between initial and blame responsibility becomes clear if we move to a higher order of abstraction. In
the theory of responsibility, two tasks are in question. The first is
the discovery of guilt. The second is the invention of guilt. Conventional behavior, custom, which in itself may even be non-moral, founds

moral responsibility. That re-arranging of our institutions in which
we engage in discussing initial responsibility gives it added moral
clout, and in so doing makes excuses pale by comparison.

VI

Excuses: For Superiors

Up until now, our viewpoint has been that of the subordinate, and
our questions have been directed towards asking how his moral stance is
affected by the job he holds. A question of equal importance concerns
the moral position of the superior. Is he, for example, to be held to
task for the actions of his subordinates?

The trials of the Axis powers at Nuremberg provide a tragic microcosm for moral responsibility in hierarchies. The viewpoint of the
subordinate was the German problem: one after another Nazi appealed to
the excuse from superior orders. The viewpoint of the superior was the
Japanese problem. Admiral Yamamoto was held responsibile for the tor-
ture of Allied prisoners of war, despite the fact that he never ordered
them to be tortured, and in fact repeatedly issued directives forbidding
the mistreatment of prisoners.[11]

What responsibility does a physician bear for a wrong committed by
a nurse under his orders? For a wrong committed independently by the
nurse?

Here is where it is important to separate legal blame-responsibility from moral blame-responsibility. The law's theory of responsibility
in part embodies factors which are foreign to morality; for example,
settledness is more important for law than for morality; so is the desire to ensure that somebody be shown to bear blame, and to ensure that
the innocent wronged party be reimbursed. In the law of torts, the general doctrine on contributory causation--in which the acts of two tort-
feasors were each necessary to produce the actionable harm--is that each
tortfeasor is responsible for the whole damage.[12] The doctrine may well
be founded upon the non-moral desiderata of the law.

It is also important in this connection to keep in mind the difference between ideal morality and the theory of blame. Ideally, a physician bears initial responsibility for the welfare of his patient, and
should be watchful of the actions of other health personnel. Absolute
surveillance, however, is clearly supererogatory. One cannot be blamed
for failing to be praiseworthy.

Provided one condition is met, our earlier discussion enables us to sidestep the question of a superior's responsibility for another's acts. That condition is that in the situation with which we are dealing blame-responsibility be a zero-sum game. In such a game, one party's loss is another party's gain.[13] This would mean for our concrete case that, to the precise extent that a nurse bears blame-responsibility for an act, a physician is absolved from guilt; to the extent that she is excused, the physician is blamed. In a zero-sum game, if you know the score of one of the players, you may deduce that of the other. If responsibility is a zero-sum game, by examining the responsibility of subordinates we may deduce the responsibility of superiors.

A number of considerations incline us to think that this condition is satisfied. There are numerous devices which we use to ensure that if one party is blamed, everyone else is free from blame. In the case of joint causation in the law, one such device is the "last clear chance rule": even if several people were negligent, liability is imposed upon the one who had the last clear chance to prevent the harm.[14] The concept mentioned earlier, the opacity of responsibility--that the chain of responsibility is broken by the action of a free agent--is also relevant in this context.

Some of the previous discussion in this paper also leans in that direction. In the case of a successful excuse founded upon a superior order, it is certainly plausible to lay the blame at the feet of the one issuing the order.

It might be objected that one who entices or coerces obedience to an immoral order is always responsible, always has some guilt. This seems to me to be a confusion. Enticing or coercing immorality are acts which are always wrong, in and of themselves, and apart from their consequences. Even an unsuccessful attempt to coerce immorality is wrong. The superior who entices or coerces obedience to an immoral order is always at fault, then, for having made this attempt. In those instances where he has offered such massive enticement or coercion as to overbear his subordinate's will, he is also guilty for the action of carrying out the immoral order: an action which he caused, although did not produce. By paying careful attention to precisely which wrongful act is in question, we may preserve the plausibility of the zero-sum condition.

The same maneuver is in place with respect to a subordinate blowing the whistle on his superior. It might be objected that the superior is in no way relieved from guilt on account of his subordinate's having wrongfully failed to blow the whistle on his conduct, thereby terminating it. But the zero-sum condition would not give that result. The superior is at fault for the wrongful action which he performs. The subordinate is at fault because he did not blow the whistle, rather than because he failed to prevent the superior's action.

The suggestion is, then, that careful parsing of the actions in question will preserve the plausibility of the zero-sum condition; so that the responsibility of superiors is deducible from that of subordinates.

VII

Conclusion

It must be stressed that everything said in this paper was written, and ought to be read, in a tentative spirit. This is not to say that I have particularly strong doubts about any of the above, still less that I have strong objections to some of the claims which I am keeping to myself. Yet the allocation of responsibility in hierarchical organizations has been so little explored that no firm conclusions should be looked for now. It should also be noted that the conclusions reached cannot serve as mathematical formulae. Judgment is required in interpreting particular situations, and in applying these conclusions.

NOTES

1   For a discussion of several major meanings of responsibility, see
    "Postscript: Responsibility and Retribution," in H. L. A. Hart,
    Punishment and Responsibility (Oxford University Press, 1963), pp.
    210-237.

2   Babylonian Talmud, Qidusin 426.

3   See I Samuel 22:18, concerning a death ordered by Saul, and the im-
    putation of murder to David in II Samuel 12:9.

4   Babylonian Talmud, Baba Mesia 106.

5   H. L. A. Hart and A. M. Honoré, *Causation In The Law* (Oxford Uni-
    versity Press, 1959), Chapters VII (tort liability) and XIII (crimi-
    nal liability).

6   Hart and Honoré, p. 324.

7   On this matter, Roman Catholic doctrine is strangely lax, as a con-
    sequence of its view that intention is relevant to the moral apprais-
    al of action, yet is something which is so wholly internal that it
    need never manifest itself in action. In Catholic doctrine, for ex-
    ample, a nurse may assist a surgeon performing an abortion, or serve
    as the anesthetist for an abortion, provided she faces very grave
    personal consequences should she refuse to do so: e.g., dismissal
    or permanent demotion. Yet abortion is considered murder. For one
    standard account of the Catholic position, see the chapter on assis-
    tance at immoral operations in Charles J. McFadden, *Medical Ethics*
    (Philadelphia: F. A. Davis Company, Sixth Edition, 1968). Catho-
    lics distinguish between formal cooperation, in which you join your
    will to the evil intention of another in obeying orders, and materi-
    al cooperation, in which you do what is requested of you while in-
    wardly not acceding to the evil intention. The former is always
    wrong, the latter may be justified in certain circumstances, as in-
    stantiated in the above example.

8   Benjamin Freedman, "A Moral Theory of Informed Consent," *Hastings
    Center Report*, vol. 5, no. 4 (1975), p. 32.

9   Robert M. Veatch, "The Generalization of Expertise," *Hastings Center
    Studies*, vol. 1, no. 2 (1973), pp. 29-40.

10 See Benjamin Freedman, "A Meta-Ethics for Professional Morality,"
    Ethics, vol. 89, no. 1 (1978), pp. 1-19.

11 See the discussion in Sanford Levinson, "Responsibility for Crimes
    of War," *Philosophy and Public Affairs*, vol. 2, no. 3 (1973),
    pp. 244-273.

12 Hart and Honoré, p. 188.

13 An example of a zero-sum game is chess, in which one player's loss
    redounds to the advantage of the other player. Monopoly is not a
    zero-sum game, since a player's loss may redound to the benefit of
    the bank.

14 Hart and Honoré, pp. 201-207.

PHYSICIAN PRIVILEGE AND ACCOUNTABILITY

LIONEL E. MCLEOD

The interest and energy demonstrated by the Institute for the Humanities in the development of a conference committed to a discussion of the powers and authorities in medical care is both admirable and timely. As both a physician and medical administrator, I offer my congratulations and my hope that this conference will take a significant step forward in a systematic examination of this particular medical care issue. It is an examination long overdue, given the charged atmosphere in which my profession functions, an atmosphere, I believe, resulting in an erosion of its major values and role in our society.

Whereas many speakers have established their pattern of thought on the problem of power and authority in medical care, my views are continuing to evolve. Many influences are unclear, inadequately focused, and outside the actual environs of the setting of the patient and the physician. I read each new article anticipating answers to the many questions on this issue, only to find more questions or elaborations of earlier questions. Only occasionally does one catch a glimpse of a path leading to improved understanding beyond the maze of conflict in which we seem to stand. To paraphrase Dr. Peter Mitchell, a Nobel prize winner in chemistry in 1978, the obscure is sometimes easily understood, the obvious is more difficult and takes much longer.

My comments will be limited to a few thoughts on the present state of affairs of physicians and a view of the direction which I believe should be taken by physicians and society. Change must be expected. In a recent annual oration of the Society of Health and Human Values, Dr. Judith Swazey predicted change in the nature of the contract between medical people and the public. Dr. Swazey stated that "the shape of that contract is still too emergent to be perceived in any but the dimmest way."[1] I hope my considerations might nudge us one small increment toward clarification of that new contract. The broader issues I leave to our more distinguished guests and colleagues.

Questioning the physician's role is frequent, becoming sharper with time, and is often hostile in nature. Criticism and questioning arise in many quarters--among politicians, health care colleagues, and

the media, to name just a few. Occasionally, organized medicine is
comforted by public polls offering views supportive of the individual
physician. The validity of such polling must be held in doubt, considering continued public interest in the failings of the medical profession. Generally, physicians singly and collectively are sensitive
to this continued criticism. To some, this is surprising, as medical
history discloses that scrutiny and criticism have always been a part
of our relationship with society at large. Humphrey Osmond, in a paper
entitled "God and the Doctor," notes that patient grumbling has a long
and venerable history.[2] Plato, for example, offered two criticisms;
one, that doctors treated slaves as carefully as they treated free men
and philosophers, actions hardly in accord with the rules of the Republic. The second criticism was that doctors treated patients, including philosophers, like slaves, a view popular amongst today's
critics of patterns of medical practice.

There are many satires depicting the practice of medicine as a
form of parasitism, extortion, or quackery. Ecclesiastes, two thousand
years ago, declared "Honor a physician with the honor due unto him for
the uses ye may have of him. For the Lord hath created him, For of the
Most High cometh healing." Treat the physician well for you may have
need of him! Yet later, Ecclesiates noted the seriousness of becoming
a patient. "He that sinneth before his Maker, let him fall into the
hands of the physician."

While of diverse origin, these widely held concerns and levelling
statements often flow from discomfort with the power and authority be-
stowed upon the physician by society and the individual patient. Dr.
John Moskop, in his paper presented at this conference, referred to
Aesculapian authority--the charismatic nature of the physician accompanied by such symbols as the white coat, the black bag, and the stethoscope. More importantly, charisma likely is perceived by those worried by potential or real pain, chronic debility, or approaching death.
Less awesomely, charisma is likely associated with the individual's
severely limited ability to assess the knowledge and competence of the
physician. As stated by Dr. Swazey, in this situation, "the patient
hands over certain freedoms to the physician to obtain benefits that
the physician offers."[3] Most of us do not relinquish freedom easily
nor without adverse reaction. Yet most experienced physicians are
aware of the therapeutic value of patient dependence and personal trust
in the physician. The charisma of the physician continues to play a

significant role in the art of medicine and should be kept in proper
perspective.

Delegation of power and authority may, in part, have another basis. Dr. W. Reich, a psychiatrist writing in Harper's, offered a further explanation.[4] Present-day criticism of the role of the psychiatrist as an agent of social control has focused on delegated power to
incarcerate individuals against their will. Criticism has been extended to the perceived power of psychiatry to influence judgments and
opinions beyond the range of psychiatric knowledge and expertise. Perhaps these criticisms are off the mark, since the real problem may be
deeper and at the heart of the physician's power and the consequent potential for abuse and error. Dr. Reich argues that the central psychiatric act, and that of any physician, is the establishment of a
diagnosis--to name, to categorize, and to explain or explain away. The
importance of this act arises from the need of each individual to know,
to understand, and to be able to explain. A diagnosis or explanation
enables us to live with ourselves and others despite a defective organ
or disease. "In powerful, self-serving, and sometimes self-deceptive
ways, we use it (the diagnosis) to alter the fright of chaos into the
comfort of the known, the burden of doubt into the pleasure of certainty, the shame of hurting others into the pride of helping them, and alter the dilemma of moral judgment into the opaque clarity of medical
truth."[5]

The strife surrounding modern medical care is eroding the central
role of the physician in the provision of medical care. While the degree of physician authority required for the provision of high quality
care varies with the physician's qualities, patient temperament, and
the nature of the disease process, it seems likely that a system of
medical care which brings about patient satisfaction will, in the main,
require a central role for the physician, reflecting medical knowledge,
skill, and understanding. Acceptance and support for that central role
will require a new and effective relationship among various professional and technical participants in view of the trends of the past. Unfortunately, it is the patient, not the professional, who has the most
to gain and the most to lose.

Perhaps a review of the common criticism and weakness of the medical model of care would be useful.

(1) *Medical care has become impersonal, hasty, fragmented, and
excessively specialty-oriented.*

Among the many factors resulting in more than a kernel of truth to this statement has been the remarkable advance in understanding of disease and its amelioration, if not control. The criticism has been trumpeted beyond the real state of medical practice, in my view. Individual experience, anecdotal evidence, and failure of the public and the profession to ensure the dissemination of information pertaining to the best use of the range of expertise have contributed to public disappointment and frustration. The considerable regional differences in style of medical practice have caused provinces and regions to offer criticism inappropriately.

Substantial emphasis on primary care by the institutions of medical education combined with a spirited interest in family practice on the part of undergraduate students will offer an answer to the need for primary and continuing care. The number of students selecting this pathway is impressive and should ensure adequate supply of primary-care physicians and contribute to the solution of physician maldistribution. The degree of this contribution is not yet clear.

The fee-for-service system does contribute to the haste and impersonal quality of an unknown percentage of patient-physician contacts. No doubt this becomes more frequent in periods when physicians perceive declining rewards for their services. On the other hand, the fee-for-service system provides clearer rewards for long hours, repetitive and uninteresting tasks, and personally trying situations. Oddly, the incentives of the fee-for-service system have not been used effectively by society to gain its objectives. Theoretically, the system could be used to address such problems as physician maldistribution, enhancement of counselling services, and the level of physician-patient communication. Despite occasional minor adjustments to the system, usually by more powerful segments of the profession, little experimentation has been attempted.

(2) *According to popular readings, too many of mankind's problems have been "medicalized."*

Many share this concern albeit not with the same vigor as Ivan Illich.[6] The physician is inadequately educated in some instances, and in others overeducated, for the wide range of concerns seeking medical solution. Medical education is intensely demanding and laden with information that must be digested and managed. Deliberate and calculated attempts are made to ensure the understanding of the physician for the impact of psychosocial factors in illness and healing. While some may

call these and other factors holistic medicine, this newly popularized
label and its related literature has added no new understandings, ideas,
or approaches to traditional concepts of patient care.

A concern of greater importance, in my view, is the limited appreciation we have for the skills and expertise of other participating pro-
essional groups, and indeed, patients themselves. A clear inhibition
to strengthening patient-care programs is our practice of educating
health care professionals in isolated clinical settings and providing
clinical preceptors not sensitive to the need for co-ordination of
patient care. The new physician is inadequately attuned to the aspirations, and often the skills, of the physiotherapist, the nutritionist,
and others. Continuing professional isolation during clinical education must perpetuate less-than-satisfactory quality of patient care.

(3) *The problem of the high cost of medical care.*

In isolation, the physician triggers the costs of medical care by
requesting hospital admission, laboratory and radiological investigation, and by prescribing treatment. In our inflationary society and in
the view of the seemingly unsaturatable sponge of patient complaint,
costs spiral. Whether the spiral exceeds that due to inflation and
population growth may be questioned. Nonetheless, the profession must
accept clear responsibility for effective and efficient use of scarce
resources and limited funding.

What is often poorly understood is the limited ability of the physician to influence the actual cost of care, the cost of equipment, and
the increasing costs of essential support staff. Indeed, appallingly,
neither the patient nor the physician in Canadian society is cognizant
of the costs of investigation and treatment. This situation courts
fiscal disaster.

Commonly, criticism of cost is focused on high-cost sophisticated
technology which is of great potential patient benefit, whereas the
massive costs of the system may be attributed to inexpensive, excessively used procedures.[7] Again, this is an area requiring re-examina-
tion of the objectives of medical education and the incentives of the
fee-for-service mechanism of payment.

The well-known increased medical requirements of the aged and
Canada's growing population of elderly citizens will add further economic stress. The potential problem is being addressed today largely
by government and hospital administrators. Only the occasional enlightened patient and unusually conscientious physician enter into the

decision-making process. A short article written in the late 1880s by
a physician described the life of the practicing physician in China.[8]
Clearly, concern for cost is not new. Part of the physician's duty,
despite the conflict of interest, was to act as an apothecary. In prescribing for the elderly, the cost was a distinct concern and related,
however subtly, to the potential benefit. Toward the conclusion of
required haggling over the value of included constituents and their
costs, a "family council is held, actually in the presence of the patient, in which the question of life and death is put, and frequently
arguments are brought forward to show that, considering the advanced
age of the patient, or the hopeless nature of the malady, it may be
better not to incur a useless expense, but quietly to allow matters to
take their course."[9] It was not uncommon for the sick man himself to
take the initiative and make the decision. An increasing number of
today's patients are prepared and often anxious to participate in clinical decision-making, though rarely with any discussion of the costs in
terms of use of resources. That latter situation may not be too distant in the future.

(4) *The alleged concentration on curative medicine and neglect
     of preventive medicine.*

The ancient Greeks stated the problem in this way: Aesculapius,
god of healing, had two daughters, Panacea (all heal), goddess of healing or clinical medicine, and Hygeia (health or hygiene), goddess of
good health and preventive medicine. Hygeia's teaching stated, "Eat
less, drink less, smoke less, fornicate less, avoid excess, exercise
prudently, or fall into the hands of my sister Panacea and her physician."

Evidence for the value of some of her admonishments is at hand,
yet public acceptance is slow and procrastination common. While the
physician may contribute to progress, the problems must be examined as
a joint venture with specialists in public education. Alliances with
the educational system must be established and despite the general protest of excessive responsibility and workloads, progress must be made.
Programs of appropriate health education must be offered a remarkably
higher priority, with teacher and health professional determining improved strategies and presenting personal habits and behaviors conducive to successful student learning.

The foregoing concerns and others result in questioning the appropriateness of the power and authority delegated by society to the

physician. Delegation, in this day, is generally accompanied by a requirement for accountability, which is expected to be offered in the
form of clear indicators that delegated powers and authority are employed properly and at a level adequately reflecting modern knowledge
and skill. While legislated responsibility and privilege partially
shelter most professions, a key ingredient for the continuation of a
mutually beneficial contract or arrangement between medicine and society is, in my view, *professional accountability*. Older dependence
upon public trust and faith is no longer sufficient. Public funding of
medical care, for the purpose of accomplishing collectively what was
impossible individually, has rapidly escalated demands for evidence of
quality control and accountability. Improved public knowledge of medical issues and the decline in support for medical myths and mystical
treatment have greatly enhanced both the demand and opportunity for
satisfactory solution. The medical profession, and its individual members, must more satisfactorily demonstrate ability to acquire medical
information in a systematic and discriminating manner and offer logical
and understandable explanations. Failure generates dissatisfaction and
distrust. The origin of this aspect of the problem, I believe, lies
both within the medical school and the prior education of the pre-medical and public school student. Excessive emphasis on information and
memory work with too little emphasis on thinking through problems and
mechanisms has dulled the curiosity and excitement required for high-
quality learning.

A second aspect to increasing public dissatisfaction is the limited visibility of the medical practitioner in the non-medical community
setting. The busy life of the practitioner has interfered with normal
contributions to society. The physician of yesteryear contributed more
willingly and effectively. The physician of today's smaller community
also may be more effective than the urban practitioner. The public
perceives that the physician has a special and valuable perspective on
today's social problems and questions the low participation. Any privileged person should understand that privilege requires attention and
careful nurturing.

As an organization, the medical profession has struggled to develop more satisfactory means of demonstrating accountability. While
today's common steps and procedures are imperfect, improvement in quality and distribution throughout society is occurring. Medical schools
and most hospitals voluntarily submit to regular external, far-reaching

review by carefully constructed survey teams. The teams of external
colleagues offer vigorous and often brutally frank criticisms and advice. Experience has resulted in improved standards against which institutions may be evaluated. Further improvement and refining is required. Progress has slowed appreciably in this time of fiscal con-
straint.

Provincial medical licensing bodies, acting under legislation,
require that tomorrow's practicing physician graduate from an accred-
ited medical school or successfully pass fairly sophisticated, albeit
imperfect written examinations. Satisfactory periods of practical
post-graduate training are required. The weakness of these requirements reflect limited medical school funding for clinical preceptors
and the inability of written examinations to efficiently and effectively evaluate the use of knowledge.

In the practice of medicine, audits and reviews of the quality of
patient care are largely limited to hospital settings, and often only
in the teaching hospital. Satisfactory performance in the hospital is
assumed to be an index of the quality of overall practice. This assumption should be critically examined, particularly in view of the
fact that a growing number of physicians practice medicine exclusively
in the office-based setting. These practitioners may rarely be exposed
to the practice of others or have reason to question their own status.
Mechanisms are needed to assess these physicians.

Programs of continuing medical education including literature reviews have become the most standard means by which the physician asses-
ses himself or herself. The use of these and related devices is becoming more widespread, though it is by no means uniform across the profession. Often it is the physician with the least need who is found to
participate regularly in continuing education. In some areas, mandatory continuing education for maintenance of practice privileges has
been required. The usefulness of mandatory attendance has been vigorously questioned as learning cannot be assured. Monitoring of competence in skills is limited exclusively to the hospital setting and
then, mainly in teaching hospitals; however the limited usefulness of
this procedure has become well known.

Computerized information on the services rendered by physicians
became readily available with the advent of medical care insurance programs. Profiles of the patterns of practice of individual physicians
are scrutinized by peers and advice offered to those physicians falling

outside the spectrum of the majority of their colleagues. Few provinces or groups seem to make full use of these opportunities largely because of the difficulties encountered in relating patterns to the quality of practice.

Presently, there is no agreement on the most reasonable means by
which the quality of physician practice may be accurately assessed.
The many methods used today could be improved and applied more widely
and more vigorously. Physician resistance to more paper, more scrutiny, more interference is widespread and justified, at least in part.
Much of the paper and scrutiny employed today has not proven productive.

A key factor for future improvement lies with the interest of medical schools in producing physicians more comfortable and co-operative
in self-assessment and the early correction of discovered deficiencies.
Significant improvement seems to be occurring. However, the concentration in the education programs on the acquisition of information
tends to override attempts to encourage so-called self-learning, self-
assessment, and peer collaboration in the evaluation of performance.
Specially designed programs are constantly threatened by the insecurity
of medical school teachers who are concerned that their particular discipline may have inadequate time and opportunity in the educational
program.

Further, the student succumbs quickly to the information-oriented
pressures of faculty and these are the same pressures the student experienced during most, if not all, of pre-medical education. Fortunately, the vagaries of clinical problems oblige the student to address
mechanisms and processes by which problems are solved.

The problem remains! The privilege of power and authority granted
physicians is an important component of the art of healing and a benefit to the patient and society. Some erosion of that arrangement with
a resulting decline in the stature of the physician likely has occurred.
However, it is worthwhile to recall the well-known rejoinder to those
who complain that the world isn't what it used to be--namely, that it
probably never was. Significant steps have been taken to improve the
credibility of the profession and to enhance its accountability. I
hope that the process of improvement continues in an accelerated manner
lest the impatience of a better-informed society irreparably damage a
valuable state of affairs.

NOTES

1 Judith P. Swazey, "Health Professionals and the Public: Toward a
   New Social Contract?", Society for Health and Human Values, Annual
   Oration, 1979.

2 Humphrey Osmond, "God and the Doctor," *New England Journal of Medicine*, 302, (1980) 555-558.

3 Swazey, "Health Professionals."

4 W. Reich, "Force of Diagnosis," *Harper's Magazine*, 260 (May, 1980),
   20.

5 *Ibid.*

6 Ivan Illich, *Limits to Medicine* (London: Marion Boyars, 1976).

7 Thomas W. Moloney and David E. Rodgers, "Medical Technology--A
   Different View of the Contentious Debate over Costs," *New England
   Journal of Medicine*, 301 (1979), 1413-1419.

8 John Williamson Palmer, "John Chapman, M.D.," in *Twelve Decades of
   Insights from the Atlantic*, Atlantic Editions, 1978.

9 *Ibid.*

HEALTH CARE

AND

PUBLIC POLICY

WHOSE RESPONSIBILITY?
PUBLIC HEALTH IN CANADA, 1919-1945

JANICE P. DICKIN MCGINNIS

"All professions," to quote George Bernard Shaw, "are conspiracies against the laity."[1] One of the distinguishing features of the twentieth century has been the institutionalization of professionalism. The ideal of the well-rounded Renaissance individual has been displaced by that of the specialist, the master of one trade and Jack of none other. Not only by its very nature but by stated intent, professionalism ousts the amateur; it removes from the general populace certain rights and opportunities to look after some of its more sophisticated needs. This limitation of individual autonomy is justified by a commitment on the part of all professions to shoulder the obligation of improved fulfillment of the relevant needs. Medical professionalization has thrived in this century because health care has been complicated by the availability of complex and expensive forms of technology that not only require expertise to make them effective, but can render lethal results in the hands of the untrained. The medical profession has fought long and hard to remove those people it considers untrained, ill-trained, or simply insufficiently trained from the field of health care. This fight, which must be recognized as more than just a selfish desire to stake a safe claim, has forged a strong link with government as the agency having jurisdiction over the legal designation of who is allowed to do what.

The medical profession needs government for more than just reasons of recognition of its prior rights to perform a certain type of task: in Canada it also depends on the public purse to provide a phenomenal amount of funds to make the practice of medicine possible. Argue as some of them may that good care is better guaranteed under a system where the doctor-patient relationship is fostered by funds actually changing hands between the consumer and the producer, Canadian doctors are dependent upon all levels of government to subsidize facilities, support personnel and equipment. Government also removes from the profession the obligation to provide for certain unprofitable classes of medical problems lumped together under the title public health. And

under the present system of health insurance, government furthermore
guarantees that each doctor will be paid for his own work, regardless
of the means of the patient. But, if government has made available to
the medical profession certain privileges, it has also made demands in
return.

The history of Canada's efforts to provide for the health of its
public between the world wars was a history of bargaining over rights
and obligations. Such negotiations were not simple bilateral affairs
conducted between the profession and the federal government. They were
complicated by the necessity also to come to terms with other levels of
government, non-professional health workers, other professions, and
the general public. As the relevant arm of the senior agency involved,
the federal health department was the focal point for much of the discussion. Particularly through its Dominion Council of Health [herein-
after DCH], it would preside over any proposed changes in Canada's
health provisions. It is obvious from studying the records of this department that privately or publicly employed members of the medical
profession were in charge of deciding what was best for the health of
Canadians. Doctors headed Canada's health departments and most of its
para-medical volunteer organizations; the profession was well represented in the House of Commons; doctors were consulted about such government
proposals as health insurance and health units. However, medical power
was not unassailable. The power of the profession vis-a-vis that of
government would be seriously weakened by the Depression, a time when
doctors were forced more and more to see government as the only possible provider of a living wage. Desperation would be relieved by the
resumption of war, but the profession, while regaining its economic
feet, would never regain its control over health decisions in this
country. Ironically this was partly due to increased sophistication in
medical technology, meaning that no physician or small group of physicians could afford to practice without government subsidies: the advance in knowledge that allowed for the individual professionalization
of medicine in the first place now curtails that individuality. But at
least as important are two related factors--the redefinition of certain
health problems as being those of a social rather than of a medical nature and the rise of professionalization in related areas, particularly
social welfare. Just as doctors gained or tried to maintain jurisdiction over specific types of activities on the grounds that they could
only properly be performed by those with specific training in that
field, by the end of World War II they were forced to confront these

restrictions raised against themselves. Responsibility for the health
of the Canadian public was not, and is not, a burden that Canadian
doctors could carry by themselves.

The breakdown of the Canadian health care system in the 1930s
demonstrated even to doctors that they could not go it alone. The solution most favored by the profession and by medically trained public
health officials was a simple one that would provide the climate doctors felt best suited to health care as they saw it. The proposed
health insurance scheme of 1945 would provide steady incomes for doctors and favorable conditions within which they could do their work.
The failure of the scheme showed not only that the Dominion and provinces could not come to terms regarding jurisdiction in health matters,
but that the definition of health care itself was changing. Volunteer
social welfare and para-medical organizations that medical men had always tried to control would win the day. Responsibility for the health
of the Canadian public would have to be shared. The social welfare reforms would go through but health insurance would not. The federal
health department itself would be subsumed into a new Department of
National Health and Welfare in which the emphasis would definitely be
on welfare.

Writing in mid-Depression, one Canadian health reformer tried to
make sense of this country's health jurisdiction by dividing it in
three.[2] The state, in which he included both the Dominion and the provinces, was in charge of legislation dealing with anti-social behavior,
prevention and control of communicable diseases, sanitation, mental
health, tuberculosis, public health education, care for poor patients,
and support of general hospitals. To private medical practice he assigned most aspects of curative medicine: maternity care, diagnosis,
care of the individual, and surgery. After making these assignments,
he was left with something he was forced to designate "the twilight
zone." In this hazy area lurked health problems of national importance
which no authority was eager to claim as wholly its own: diagnosis and
treatment of tuberculosis and venereal disease, "maternity and infant
care," immunization, and vaccination. Obviously, packaging health care
according to arbitrary ideas of who should have power over what, was
leaving the job half done, if that. Separation of public health and
medical care, particularly, had been impossible to justify since, as
one prominent Canadian health figure put it, "Pasteur's work revealed
man as the reservoir of his own infections."[3] Provisions for

tuberculosis control in Canada will illustrate the problems of dividing
responsibility for health. A high standard of public health (the preserve of the Dominion) necessitated a low TB rate. However, an important way of preventing the disease was to treat its victim (the preserve of the medical profession), preferably in hospitals (the preserve
of the provinces). In order to prevent possible relapse of an arrested
case, job counselling and health education (the preserves, by default,
of the voluntary organizations) were needed. This confusion had arisen
in spite of repeated attempts to rationalize responsibility for health
care in Canada.

I

Federal and Provincial Health Jurisdiction

When the British North America Act was drawn up in 1867, responsibility for health was given short shrift. At that time, health care
was considered a family, or at most, a community affair.[4] The Act contains precisely two references to health matters. One assigns exclusively to the federal sphere responsibility for "Quarantine and the
Establishment and Maintenance of Marine Hospitals"; the other assigns
exclusively to the provinces "The Establishment, Maintenance, and
Management of Hospitals, Asylums, Charities, and Eleemosynary Institutions in and for the Provinces, other than Marine Hospitals." Failure
to make more precise references to public health was due neither to intent nor oversight. It simply was not a matter of any import: the term
"public health" itself was not even yet in vogue.[5] What grew up in this
vacuum of neglect was a system wherein individual medical practitioners
looked after individual care, the provinces and municipalities provided
hospital beds, and the federal government confined itself largely to
the control of environmental conditions. By 1896, responsibility for
health matters needed more precise legal definition, and the BNA Act
was reinterpreted, placing the great majority of previously unmentioned
functions under the jurisdiction of the provinces.[6] The placing of
health in the new class of provincial responsibilities would be disputed
for at least the next half century. A document produced at the end of
the Great War to support the establishment of a federal Department of
Health interpreted the BNA Act to mean that all new matters, particularly health, fell rightly under federal responsibility.[7] An article
by a prominent public health official that was published in 1940 and

reprinted in 1962 made the same argument.[8] But, all arguments aside,
the federal government would always act under the assumption that the
reverse was the case. Newton W. Rowell, when introducing in the House
of Commons in 1919 the act establishing the first federal Department of
Health, added to the confusion by stating that in regard to health matters

> I think the provinces clearly have jurisdiction,
> but the Federal Government also has jurisdiction.
> It seems to be a case of both having jurisdiction....[9]

However, the Dominion would always assume that the provinces had prior
rights and prior responsibility. At first it would accept this position regretfully; one federal official complained to another in 1919
about "the complication caused by Canada having left all matters relating to health to the Provinces, which we can now see was a great
mistake."[10] But by the early years of the Depression, the Dominion
would accept the designation gratefully, producing numerous studies to
show that it was up to the provinces to cover the serious shortfall in
provisions for Canadian health care exaggerated by the economic emergency.[11] The Department would, by and large, restrict itself to two
types of health activities that were a natural outgrowth of the few
activities, scattered among various departments,that the federal government had always performed in public health. The first type of activity
had to do with quarantine, in the broadest possible sense. The federal
government kept sick people out of the country, germs out of certain
water supplies, adulterated food out of Canadian larders, and dangerous drugs out of Canadian medicine chests. The second type of activity
involved co-ordination of health activity in general in the country.
This it hoped to accomplish largely through the publication of great
quantities of instructive literature and through twice-yearly meetings
of the Dominion Council of Health attended by all provincial deputy
ministers of health and five interested laypersons. When the Department did choose to take a more active role, such as in the fields of
venereal disease and child welfare, it usually did so by subsidizing
work done by the provinces or by the two other groups taking responsibility for Canadian health, the medical profession and various volunteer
organizations.[12]

It is difficult to make similar generalizations about the health
activities of the various provinces. Differences would be vast, as
health provisions in the individual provinces depended "too largely"
on economic conditions in those provinces.[13] At the time of the

establishment of the federal department in 1919, all provinces had some
sort of health board, and in 1917, New Brunswick had set up the first
ministry of health in the British Empire. Under each of these boards
there was a plethora of local and municipal health boards that had only
recently, and only in some cases, begun to grow into more than stop-gap
emergency organizations originally established to deal with the epidemic
diseases of the eighteenth and nineteenth centuries, notably typhus and
cholera. Most provincial boards concentrated on the fields of quarantine, laboratory service, and sanitary inspection. Some branched out
into child welfare (Ontario) and "publicity" (Quebec, Ontario, Alberta,
and British Columbia). Nova Scotia, Quebec, Manitoba, and Saskatchewan
collected vital statistics. No province, with the possible exception of
Saskatchewan, seemed to have a conscious plan in mind. The annual report of the ground-breaking New Brunswick health ministry did not include anything on areas outside of St. John and Fredericton. Prince Ed-
ward Island issued no annual health report at all. The practice of all
provinces was simply to address themselves to new problems as their
solution became urgent.[14]

The federal and provincial health departments would grow up together, and the agency meant to act as their guardian was the Dominion Council of Health, established in conjunction with the federal Department in
1919. The DCH had, in fact, no power to do anything. This had been
written into its charter from the outset[15] and was apparently one reason
for its appeal. Its favored function was to be a think tank where Canada's top health officials and a few chosen laypersons could talk over
health ideas twice a year. It was hoped that in this way the DCH would
be an organ that, although it might not be able to force change, would
at least have some influence. One Dominion health minister stated his
faith in the Council by arguing that it was impossible that all the
hours of talk "did not produce some good."[16] But, in truth, many of
those hours of talk took the DCH directly up blind alleys. Examples of
matters on which it had spent considerable time to little or no avail
were treatment facilities for drug addicts; uniform provincial regulations for disinfectants; co-operation in halting a scheme, potentially
dangerous to human life, to manufacture a virus to commit germ warfare
against rats; cleanliness standards for converted materials used for
stuffing upholstery, bedding, toys, etc.; co-operation among the provinces for the safe shipment of deceased persons across provincial bor-
ders; and, a very important issue, inter-provincial organization of reciprocal care for sufferers from TB and other dangerous communicable

diseases moving from one province to another. The Council also spent considerable time on more profitable discussions on maternal and infant hygiene, venereal disease, health insurance, the establishment of clinics, quarantine, immigration medical inspection, and other matters vital to Canadian public health.[17]

Still, despite the mass of good information and informed opinion exchanged, co-ordination of health care in each of the provinces did not develop. Neither did co-ordination between the Dominion and any of the individual provinces. What was needed to bring both about was money and legislation, and the DCH had control over neither. By the start of the Depression, provisions still differed fundamentally from one province to another. Each province might take care of areas such as collection of vital statistics, control of communicable diseases, treatment and control of venereal disease and tuberculosis, maternal hygiene, pre-school and school hygiene, food and milk control, community sanitation, sanitary engineering, health education, cancer control, heart disease clinics, industrial hygiene, mental hygiene and mental hospitals, inspection of hospitals, dental services, and training schools for nurses.[18] These did not add up to a co-ordinated health program for any province, nor did they, when added to what the Dominion was doing, add up to a coordinated health program for the country.

II

The Medical Profession

After the federal and provincial governments, the major organized body concerned with Canadian health care was the medical profession. One of the problems the federal health department would have in dealing with the profession was the conviction of that group that the Department was at least partly a creature of its own invention. The Canadian Medical Association [hereinafter CMA] had certainly lobbied for a federal health department for some years prior to its actual establishment[19] and the entire profession was congratulated in the House of Commons for "having, as a result of their consistent labors, at last secured a Public Health Act that. . . meets with the approval of everybody."[20] Not everyone was happy about the hold Canadian doctors had over the delivery of health care and were expected to have over the new Department. Articles in the public press accused the profession of pressuring for its establishment simply to gain official representation of its views at the federal government level and Christian Scientists, fearing that the new

Department would force them to go to doctors, launched a write-in campaign.[21] If it were not precisely true that the profession had created
and would control the Department, doctors--particularly as represented
by the CMA--would exercise considerable influence. Doctors held a special status in the eyes of most of the Canadian population, of the politicians, and certainly of Department officials. They were the experts
and the healers. It was taken for granted that their needs and wishes
must be taken into account when it came to reforming any part of the
Canadian health care system.

Another factor that militated in favor of special treatment of the
medical profession by most health officials and Ministers was that most
of these gentlemen were themselves members of the medical profession.
They had profited from the same training, subscribed to the same ideals,
and supported the same methods as the group with which they were to ne-
gotiate, if not actually to direct. One doctor, later to become for a
short period Minister of Health, stood in the House of Commons to claim
that "if you look over the history of health matters throughout the
world, you will find that there has been no advance in sanitation or
public health that medical men were not foremost in helping forward."[22]
Another doctor, while actually serving as Minister, referred to the
medical profession as "that splendid branch of humanity."[23] To be fair,
they were not alone in this adulation. Non-professionals also stood in
the House to make similar votes of confidence in Canadian doctors.[24]
Nowhere would doctors' special status be more apparent than in the attitude of Parliament and the Department towards the prosecution of physicians suspected or even guilty of drug offences. It was considered
not quite fair to use the evidence of either decoys or addicts to gain
a conviction against a member of the medical profession.[25] It was asked
that doctors who were addicted themselves be given more leeway and not
be prosecuted even if they supplied narcotics to children. Due to their
addiction, they could not be considered responsible for their acts, and
the Department should not treat them the same as any other criminal involved with narcotics.[26] Although the Narcotics Division saw that
charges were laid against some medical offenders, it did so reluctant-
ly.[27] Instead, the chief of the Division preferred to obtain from the
offender a guarantee that he would "take a cure."[28]

In addition to this deference to the medical man as a special person, there was a tendency on the part of the Department to use the medical profession as a source of objective opinion in matters in which it

could not possibly be objective. Because of this, the profession did
have some control over Departmental activities and policy--never official control, but control all the same. This power was most prominently
put into force when it came to safeguarding the predominant place of
doctors in the health care delivery system. Mid-wives especially were
a constant thorn in the side of the medical profession. Considered
"pretty dangerous individuals owing to their fixed ideas,"[29] mid-wives
existed in Canada for the simple reason that they were needed, particularly in areas where doctors had chosen, for reasons of isolation or
unprofitability, not to settle. The profession worried that mid-wives
might give inferior care but also that they might siphon off an ever-
increasing part of doctors' business. For much the same reasons, the
profession resisted the professionalization of optometrists, chiroprac-
tors, osteopaths, and homeopaths, as well as faith healers with no pre-
tense to training at all.[30] It also sought to reduce the flow of foreign doctors into Canada, on the grounds that there was no room for
them, except in certain parts of the west, due to large graduating
classes from Canadian medical schools.[31] Provincial as well as federal
governments helped the profession to protect its own monopoly in this
field.[32] The Department and the profession also worked hand in hand in
other matters. It is true that the profession did not always get its
way,[33] and that the Department also solicited opinions from other bodies which were not capable of taking objective stands,[34] but time after
time the Department asked for and took into account the advice of Canadian doctors on matters that involved their own regulation. And when
medical care systems broke down under the force of the Depression, the
first reaction of the Department was to leave new initiative for change
in the hands of the Canadian Medical Association.

III

Voluntary Organizations

The remaining group shouldering responsibility for Canadian health
was comprised of the voluntary organizations. Certain of these organizations, like the Victorian Order of Nurses, the Canadian Tuberculosis
Association, and the Health League of Canada, had received grants from
the federal Department ever since it was established. However, aside
from administering such grants, the federal health authorities seemed a
little at a loss as to how they were to deal with these independent organizations, and the organizations themselves had different ideas about

what they expected from the Department. The Canadian Red Cross, for
example, asked the Department for some sort of official recognition,
but the Department only urged it and similar agencies to organize themselves under the aegis of the Canadian Public Health Association which,
while independent, had close ties with the Department.[35] At the same
time, members of the Department, the DCH, and the provincial health
boards all were trying to gain control over Canada's child welfare societies insisting that they, as medical men, should act as "parents" to
these paramedical organizations. Their advances were firmly spurned.
These groups saw themselves as dealing with problems that transcended
purely medical solutions. They would co-operate but would not be
"driven."[36] Throughout the 1920s, Canada's non-governmental health
agencies were left pretty much to their own devices, some receiving
grants and others having leading health officials sitting on their executives.

There was another--a foreign--organization that gained considerable power during this period. Starting in 1925, the Rockefeller Foundation began funding, unlike certain agencies, activities that were
squarely within the health field: establishment of schools of hygiene;
fellowships for medical health officers, public health nurses and personnel from government health departments; full-time country health
units in some provinces; home nursing; and education regarding nutrition and health practices. It, too, made grants to various voluntary
agencies.[37] The provincial representatives on the DCH were not happy
about this invasion of their territory. They asked the federal government to provide money to displace the Foundation on the grounds that
"we had better be the 'mother' rather than the Rockefeller people."[38]
The change in attitude to the Rockefeller Foundation wrought by the
economic exigencies of the Depression illustrates the general change in
attitude towards all the non-governmental agencies. By 1936, the federal Deputy Minister of Health would be forced to admit that: "We, as
a Dominion Department, could bury our pride sufficiently to accept
money, if we could get it from him [Rockefeller]."[39] All Canadian governments would accept and expect strong back-up from the volunteer societies during the 1930s.

IV

Effect of the Depression upon Health Care Organization

Despite the high hopes that had led to the establishment of the
federal Department in 1919, public health made little progress in Canada in the 1920s. The federal Department itself had lost ground by
the end of the decade and had been amalgamated with Soldiers' Civil
Re-establishment to form the new Department of Pensions and National
Health where the emphasis would certainly be on the former. By 1930,
all levels of government in Canada spent only a total of seventeen
million dollars on prevention while the total expenditures on the
treatment of illness were nearly $273,000,000.[40] Health care in Canada
was obviously still built on the cornerstone of personal ameliorative
treatment of the individual. The Canadian health system was unprepared
for a situation in which a vast number of Canadians could not pay for
this care. It had so far functioned by roughly dividing responsibility
among the Dominion (literature, some health care, and some funding),
the provinces and municipalities (hospitals, some clinics, school
health programs, and so forth), the voluntary organizations (fund-rais-
ing, propaganda, care of certain special and indigent cases) and the
medical profession (medical care, including some unpaid care). The
economic emergency would cause increased call for free care at the
same time as it would cut back the funds available to all these bodies.
At first health problems would be ignored while everyone got on with
the more pressing problems of general poor relief, but by mid-decade,
when it was beginning to appear that hard times could last forever,
attempts were made to find long-term solutions. The federal government
constantly waved the BNA Act, saying it was barred by the constitution
from becoming involved. All provinces went ahead with some sort of
medical relief in the form of health units, municipal doctor systems,
and direct subsidies to the medical profession in return for service to
the poor. Such schemes were not drawn up solely with the interests of
the needy public in mind; they were also designed to help the medical
profession. Finally, by the end of the Depression, the Dominion would
bow to the constant calls made on it to provide some long-term solution.
It, too, would consider the doctors.

Doctors became alarmed at the effect of the Depression on health
care in Canada not just because of their role as safeguarders of Canadian health but because they were the sellers of a service that could

be afforded by an ever smaller number of consumers. Like everyone else
in the country, doctors needed work--or at least paid work. It was
said that, in the search for a living wage, some doctors had been
forced to take jobs as taxi drivers and manual laborers; others had
gone on relief.[41] It was also said that, in an attempt to carry on
their work, some doctors had mortgaged their possessions, unable as
they were to collect fees from their destitute patients.[42] By mid-
decade, some doctors in the Winnipeg area banded together to attempt to
force the municipal government to shoulder some of the load when it
came to free medical service for the poor. Those involved signed a
pledge refusing to give free care to those receiving relief from the
city. Doctors wanted payment.[43] This was a move dangerously close to
strike action, something that had been anathema to the medical mind.
However, it was admittedly unfair to the profession to ask them to provide free service. After all, no other profession was asked to do so,
nor were manufacturers expected to supply free goods. However, while
they were eager to be paid, doctors also worried about the fate the
profession might suffer if it delivered itself even partially to state
subsidization. As one editorial in the *Canadian Public Health Journal*
asked, "Is medical relief the fore-runner of state medicine?"[44] But it
was clearly time for the profession to act and doctors realized it.[45]
In 1933, the Saskatchewan representative to the DCH urged such action,
warning that "it behooves the medical profession to be prepared with
some fairly definite leadership, while public opinion [is] still flu-
id."[46]

One of the problems with medical initiative in this field was that
fear of regulation on the part of the doctors would hamper any negotiation of a system of subsidized medicine satisfactory to both the state
and the profession.[47] One doctor admitted in the House of Commons that
the characteristic individualism pervading the medical profession
meant that it had "probably not advanced or kept step with the organization of other fields of activity."[48] Doctors were used to being controlled by other doctors, from training school on, and worried that the
relegation of even part of this control to another body would destroy
individual initiative and the much-advertised "personal element" in
doctor-patient relations.[49] The party taking the other side in the negotiations would also have trouble with the concept of regulating the
profession. While it could be argued that doctors knew little about
public health,[50] it could not be argued that public health officials
were similarly ignorant of the doings of private physicians. They were

doctors and they were active in the profession. This was especially
true of the federal Department. According to the constitution of the
Canadian Medical Association, two members of the CMA General Council
had to be officials of the Department, one of whom must be the Deputy
Minister.[51] It went without saying that the profession would have
strong influence on any government decision as to its fate.[52] The
solutions meant to alleviate not only the suffering of impoverished,
unhealthy Canadians but the financial woes of physicians were introduced under the shadow of uneasy negotiation. The scheme eventually
settled upon by the federal government--compulsory health insurance--
would suffer from too close concern for the feelings of the profession
and then would suffer the final indignity of being rejected by that
profession when it felt it no longer needed it.

V

The Proposal of Health Insurance

Health insurance was not a new idea. It had first been introduced
in Germany in 1883 and by 1936 had been legislated in twenty-five
countries.[53] In Canada, British Columbia had considered such a plan
immediately after the Great War and had enacted one in the mid-1930s.
At that point it had run into opposition from the business community,
which said it could not pay the percentage of costs expected from it,
and the medical profession, which objected to the fact that the very
poor would not be covered and therefore would still come to doctors
for unpaid care. Alberta also passed a similar law in the mid-1930s,
but this one disappeared with a change of government.[54] The federal
health department had considered various schemes for health insurance
since the late 1920s and in 1934, desperate for paid work, the Canadian
Medical Association released the report of its Committee on Economics
which gave unofficial approval to health insurance.[55] Although Canadian health insurance studies were started with an eye to dealing with
the problems of the Depression, the interruption of a war did not kill
the discussion. It was variously feared that an epidemic would follow
the Second World War as it had the First, that depression would return,
for which it would be best to be prepared, and that failure to provide
for the health of Canadians might foster revolutionary fervor. The
federal government set up the Advisory Committee on Health Insurance
in February 1942 and, after hours of hearings, it released its report

just over a year later.[56] Its proposals would appear as part of the
slate of social security measures the Dominion and provinces would ne-
gotiate in the immediate post-war period.

The health reform proposals were based on the idea that there was
a fixed pool of ill health in the community which could be measured by
adding up all health expenditures in the country in a recent year. A.
E. Grauer had come up with the figure of $253,113,671 or $24.69 per
capita for the year 1931 when he was preparing his report for the
Rowell-Sirois Commission on Dominion-Provincial Relations in the late
1930s. The Advisory Committee on Health Insurance settled on a sum
very close to this: $250,000,000 or $21.60 per person. One hundred
million dollars of the needed funds were to come from individual contributions, an equal amount from Dominion general revenues and the last
fifty million dollars from Dominion income tax. The $21.60 allotment
per person per year was to cover doctors' fees, hospital care, nursing
services, dental care, pharmaceuticals, and laboratory services. General practitioner service was allowed six dollars per year and other
doctors' services--in the form of consultant, specialist, or surgical
attention--were allowed an additional $3.50. This meant that the medi-
cal profession was to receive nearly forty-five per cent of the funds.
Dentists, by comparison, were allowed only $3.60 and all nursing ser-
vices only $1.75 per annum. All laboratory services were expected to
cost no more than sixty cents and hospitalization was to be provided for
less than four dollars a year per person. In addition to the funds to
enact these health insurance proposals, there was a planning and organization grant to aid the individual provinces in introducing their separate but equal schemes and in training necessary personnel; health
grants for the fields of tuberculosis, mental health, venereal disease,
physical fitness, special investigations in public health and professional training for physicians, engineers, nurses, and sanitary inspec-
tors; and financial assistance for the construction of hospitals. To
obtain Dominion money, each province had to make promises and cash commitments of its own.[57] It was an ambitious scheme--too ambitious.

VI

The Failure of Health Insurance

The scheme failed partly because of its own defects. Actuarially,
its calculations were open to attack. Affirmations that "public health
is dirt cheap"[58] were simply not true. As one study pointed out,

insurance allowed people to make greater demands on existing facilities
and this brought ever increasing costs.[59]   This was not a matter of patients or doctors abusing the system, as some feared, simply a matter
of people being able to do precisely what the plan intended--to have
their physical complaints treated. If enacted, the plan would also
have led to stress of epidemic proportions on existing facilities. Although the whole package included grants to help the provinces expand
their facilities, there would, of necessity, have been a time lag before this could be performed. In the meantime, the call on hospitals
and professionals would be overwhelming.[60]   One official estimated that
three times the number of dentists would be needed immediately.[61]   The
scheme could also be attacked for leaning too far in favor of doctors.
Physicians were to receive a portion of the premiums that was out of
all proportion with actual health care costs.

The medical profession was involved in the government study from
the first. The Canadian Medical Association had started its own studies into health insurance in 1929.[62]   The Depression had increased the
profession's interest in what might prove to be the answer to doctors'
acute problems of getting payment for their services. It is possible
that the war also added to their fears. Not only was there the spectre
of another post-war depression, there was the more tangible possibility
that medical officers would return from the war only to find their patients dispersed and their practices defunct, as had happened at the
end of World War I.[63]   Canadians certainly had no objection to doctors
being guaranteed a living wage. A traditionally rather radical member
of the House of Commons stressed the need for provision of health care
because "first, there is the urgent need of those who are ill, and,
second, the doctor."[64]   A propaganda pamphlet on health insurance circulated to the armed forces asked if it were fair for doctors to provide service with little or no hope of remuneration.[65]   But, although
doctors might want some government support, they strongly feared concomitant government control of their traditionally independent profession.[66]   They feared that, since politicians represented the consumers
of medical service, there would be a tendency on the part of these politicians to ignore the rights of the producers (the doctors) in order
to please their constituents.[67]   Therefore, although they were willing
in the end to let the government take over all financial aspects, they
still wanted control not only over the types of services to be provided
but also over the fees to be paid.[68]   The Department had a long tradition of close co-operation with the Canadian Medical Association. This

is not to say the relationship was not without strife. For example,
when the CMA asked the Department in 1929 if the latter cared to join
the profession in an investigation of health insurance rather than vice
versa, a federal official complained that it was endeavoring "to run
away with the whole show."[69]

The Department would not follow the advice of one Member of Parliament that the doctors should be encouraged to formulate a scheme of
their own liking, thereby avoiding any refusal on their part to participate.[70] But the Deputy Minister of Pensions and National Health
would assure the CMA that the officials of the Department "do our utmost to maintain at every turn the interests of the practitioners of
Canada as well as organized medicine."[71] The Department did not act
so closely with other bodies on legislation respecting them. When suggestions were put that an advisory board of representatives from the
relevant industries be established to advise the Department on legislation regarding the manufacture of food and drugs, one senior Department
official argued that: "It does not appear logical that the Government
of Canada should hand over the privilege of making laws to a group of
individuals who have their own ends to serve."[72] Now, the Department
was collaborating closely with the Canadian Medical Association--so
closely, in fact, that the Royal College of Physicians and Surgeons of
Canada was rather irritated[73]--on a matter that certainly could serve
the profession's ends.[74] The CMA was called in, confidentially, to
discuss health insurance even before the first draft was taken before
the DCH.[75] By 1942, the liaison was official and public: it was announced in the *Canadian Medical Association Journal* that the Department
would co-operate closely with the CMA's Committee of Seven.[76] As before, negotiations did not always go smoothly. At one point, the CMA
Committee set up its own headquarters in the Chateau Laurier and demanded that the head of the federal committee wait upon it rather than
the other way around.[77] And the CMA was not always constant in its
support of the proposed measures. In 1943, the CMA Council approved
health insurance in principle,[78] and the support of its past president
was lauded in the House of Commons.[79] After the Dominion lost a jurisdictional dispute with the provinces, however, and the profession faced
negotiation with nine separate political bodies, the CMA withdrew its
support.[80]

In the end, Canada's health insurance plan was wrecked on the
shoals of Dominion-provincial relations. The provinces felt the Dominion was asking them to give up too much in the way of power and taxes

in return for subsidization of health insurance. The federal government might have pushed matters had it been sure it could afford the scheme itself.[81] Still, the BNA Act might have been overcome and the money found had conditions been different. But the truth of the matter was that other reforms took precedence over health insurance. Unemployment insurance and family allowances simply seemed more pressing and widespread in their benefits. It could be argued that, whereas health insurance would not improve prosperity--except perhaps for those employed by the health care industry--a system of welfare payments (including unemployment benefits and family allowances) would improve the standard of health.[82] As the Director of Public Health of Montreal pointed out in a speech before the Health League of Canada in Toronto in October, 1942: "One of the reasons for the relatively low level of public health in Canada is certainly that there are altogether too many families with insufficient incomes."[83] Although it was still true that a serious illness, especially a chronic one, could wreck even the most carefully planned and comfortably cushioned budget,[84] even the Director of Health Insurance Studies stated in 1933 that "[personally], I would prefer to see unemployment insurance established before health insurance."[85]

VII

Conclusion

Canada established its first federal department of health in 1919 to bring order to health care in this country. The reform was ineffective for several reasons. One was that it was not strong enough to fulfil even contemporary needs. In keeping with the ideal of individualism inherent in the medical profession controlling public and private health care, the federal department could advise but not control in many fields under its jurisdiction. Attempts to strengthen control were further thwarted by the anomalies of the BNA Act and the very real fact that neither federal nor provincial governments had sufficient funds to force acceptance of their own priorities. Voluntary groups with a leaning towards social welfare solutions were undermining medical power by tapping different sources of funds and applying them in a manner that sometimes by-passed medical solutions altogether. The role of medicine, in turn, was affected by changes in the twentieth century. Just as that profession had argued for hegemony over certain matters on the grounds that special training was needed, social welfare professionals could now use the same argument. Neither could medical professionals simply expand their training to upgrade their qualifications and thereby continue as experts in fields they had previously dominated. The boom in medical technology throughout the twentieth century has made it difficult for medical professionals to maintain a well-rounded grasp of matters considered unequivocally medical, let alone matters to do with such fields as social science, economics or--that discipline considered part of the proper training of any nineteenth-century doctor--the humanities.

Health care in Canada did not react quickly to this change in conditions. Despite the fact that public health, even in the limited manner in which it was defined, failed to make headway during the 1920s and broke down disastrously during the 1930s, it took the catalyst of the Second World War to effect true efforts for reform. However, the reform proposed was one that looked to the past--to shoring up the old system rather than to re-forming the Canadian health care system for the future. It would fail for a complicated set of reasons but not least of all because, as it was envisioned, it was an idea whose time had passed. With it had passed the place of the medical doctor as the expert on all facets of human life that had effect upon a broadly defined concept of individual health. The expertise and advice of economists and sociologists, rather than that of doctors, were now sought after in the solution of certain social problems, and the more direct aspects of care were moving more into the hands of social workers and other health professionals.

Health insurance had been devised under the assumption that health problems were amenable to medical treatment and that medical treatment should be supervised by doctors. The medical profession and medically trained public health officials had combined to come up with the best possible solution they could envision under the circumstances. The fact that they were out of date was not only demonstrated by the failure of the plan but by other changes. In 1935, a lawyer, not a doctor, was named Minister of Pensions and National Health, a fact much remarked upon in the House.[86] In 1944, the federal department was changed to National Health and Welfare and the term health was only kept in the title after some fighting from health groups.[87] With the end of the war, the health professions would find that they no longer negotiated with Canada's governments on a doctor-to-doctor basis but through other professionals--lawyers and economists.[88] In 1978, a minor official of the Department of National Health and Welfare remarked that, in recent years, "doctors have done very badly" within the administration of the Department.[89]   Meanwhile, the welfare aspects have grown by leaps and bounds. In a way it is the revenge of those voluntary organizations that the medical profession tried to control in the 1920s. While the 1930s had been a hard time for an established profession like medicine, it had been a time of growth for those interested in welfare. Post-war recognition and funding would allow them to build on the base they had established for themselves during the Depression. One cannot say that the medical profession has done badly since 1945, but it has cer-tainly lost the hegemony it once had over all provisions for the well-being of the individual.

NOTES

1 George Bernard Shaw, *The Doctor's Dilemma* (Baltimore: Penguin Books, 1965), p. 116. Originally published in 1913. The character who speaks this line in the "tragedy" is Sir Patrick Cullen, "a middle-aged doctor."

2 Allon Peebles, "The State and Medicine," *Canadian Journal of Economics and Political Science*, 2 (Nov. 1936), 476.

3 Grant Fleming, "The Relationship of Public Health to Medical Care," *Canadian Public Health Journal* [hereinafter *CPHJ*], 25 (Oct. 1934), 461.

4 Peter Aucoin, "Federal Health Care Policy," in *Issues in Canadian Public Policy*, ed. by G. Bruce Doern and V. Seymour Wilson (Toronto: Macmillan, 1974), p. 55.

5 R. D. Defries, ed., *The Development of Public Health in Canada* (Toronto: Canadian Public Health Association, 1940), p. vii.

6 Anthony H. Birch, *Federalism, Finance and Social Legislation in Canada, Australia and the United States* (Toronto: Oxford University Press, 1955), p. 73.

7 Public Archives of Canada [hereinafter PAC], RG 29, Records of the Department of National Health and Welfare, vol. 19, file 10-3-1, part 2, Report to the Vice-Chairman of the War Committee of the Cabinet on the Establishment of a Federal Department of Public Health, 25 Oct. 1918, p. 28.

8 K. F. Brandon, "Public Health in Upper Canada," in Defries, *The Development of Public Health in Canada*, p. 65, and in *The Federal and Provincial Health Services in Canada*, 2nd ed., ed. by R. D. Defries (Toronto: Canadian Public Health Association, 1962), p. 139.

9 Canada, House of Commons, *Debates* [hereinafter Commons, *Debates*], 1919, p. 1170.

10 PAC, RG 29, vol. 19, file 10-3-1, part 2, letter from Francis H. Gisborne, Parliamentary Counsel to Frederick Montizambert, Director General of Public Health, Department of Immigration and Colonization, 10 Jan. 1919.

11 PAC, RG 29, vol. 23, file 21-1-1 contains several memos produced to back up assertions of provincial responsibility.

12 For a detailed account of federal activities in health see Janice P. Dickin McGinnis, "From Health to Welfare. Federal Government Policies Regarding Standards of Public Health for Canadians, 1919-1945," unpublished Ph.D. dissertation, University of Alberta, 1980, chapters 1-4.

13 G. H. Castleden, Commons, *Debates*, 1940, p. 641.

14 See Defries, ed., *The Development of Public Health in Canada*, p. vii, and *The Federal and Provincial Health Services in Canada*, p. 136-7. Also see the section on Administration of Public Health under Provincial Governments in PAC, RG 29, vol. 19, file 10-3-1, part 2, Report to the Vice-Chairman of the War Committee..., p. 24-25c.

15 N. W. Rowell, Commons, *Debates*, 1919, p. 1173.

16 J. H. King, Commons, *Debates*, 1929, p. 2816.

17 See PAC, MG 28, Records of the Dominion Council of Health [herein-after DCH Minutes], starting Oct. 1919, microfilm reel C-9814 on.

18 PAC, RG 29, vol. 23, file 21-1-1, Activities of Dominion and Provincial Departments of Health in Respect to Overlapping, p. 2.

19 See correspondence in PAC, RG 29, vol. 19, file 10-3-1, part 1.

20 Francis H. Keefer, Commons, *Debates*, 1919, p. 1378.

21 *Ibid.*, 1919, p. 1179 (R. J. Manion), p. 1372 (W. D. Cowan), and p. 1378 (F. H. Keefer). See correspondence in PAC, RG 29, vol. 19, file 10-3-1, part 2.

22 R. J. Manion, Commons, *Debates*, 1919, p. 1179.

23 Murray MacLaren, *ibid.*, 1932-33, p. 3118.

24 For example, F. H. Keefer, *ibid.*, 1919, p. 1378.

25 J. P. Howden, *ibid.*, 1934, p. 1679; Peter McGibbon, J. P. Howden, and Robert K. Anderson, *ibid.*, 1928, pp. 4052-7.

26 Arthur E. Ross, *ibid.*, 1929, p. 2978.

27 For example, Canada, *Report of the Department of Pensions and National Health, 1931*, p. 79.

28 PAC, RG 29, vol. 236, file 324-1-2, part 1, letter from Col. C. H. L. Sharman to Dr. A. Proctor, registrar of the College of Physicians and Surgeons, British Columbia, 19 March 1930. In 1941 he estimated that 120 Canadian doctors had benefited from this option over the past twelve years. *Ibid.*, vol. 237, file 324-1-2, part 4, letter from Sharman to H. J. Anslinger, Commissioner of Narcotics, Treasury Department, Washington, D. C., 3 Feb. 1941.

29 J. A. Amyot, Deputy Minister of the Department of Health, Canada. PAC, DCH Minutes, 8th meeting, 19-21 June 1923, p. 11.

30 PAC, DCH Minutes, 14th meeting, 26-28 Oct. 1926, pp. 38-9. See PAC, RG 29, vol. 183, file 302-6-3 and file 302-6-4, part 1. PAC, RG 29, vol. 39, file 35-2-4, part 1, letter to Department from Dame Veuve Pierre Sicard of Jolliette, P. Q., 1 Feb. 1927. James H. Gray, *The Roar of the Twenties* (Toronto: Macmillan, 1975), p. 224.

31 See correspondence, PAC, RG 29, vol. 184, file 302-6-10, part 1 on reciprocal recognition of medical qualifications.

32 PAC, DCH Minutes, 3rd meeting, 25-26 Oct. 1920, p. 18. Paul Victor
    Collins, "The Public Health Policies of the United Farmers of Al-
    berta Government, 1921-1935" (unpublished M.A. thesis, University
    of Western Ontario, 1969), pp. 35-9. See correspondence in PAC, RG
    29, vol. 183, file 302-6-3.

33 For example, regarding relaxation of narcotics restrictions on
    prescriptions by doctors. PAC, RG 29, vol. 858, file 20-C-33,
    part 1, memo from the CMA to the Minister of Pensions and National
    Health [early 1935?].

34 For example, the Canadian Pharmaceutical Manufacturers Association
    and individual manufacturing firms. C. G. Power, Commons, *Debates*,
    1939 (1st session), pp. 822-3.

35 See PAC, RG 29, vol. 861, file 20-C-46, part 1, correspondence be-
    tween Canadian Red Cross and the Department, October 1919. See
    discussions regarding voluntary organizations in DCH Minutes, 2nd
    meeting, May 1920; 3rd meeting, Oct. 1920 and 6th meeting, June
    1922.

36 See the discussion in PAC, DCH Minutes, 3rd meeting, 25-26 Oct.
    1920, pp. 11-13.

37 T. B. Windross, "More than One Thousand Lives Saved Annually by
    Alberta Health Services," Calgary *Herald*, 21 July 1934. Defries,
    The Development of Public Health in Canada, p. ix. PAC, RG 29,
    vol. 97, file 156-2-4, letter from C. M. Hincks of the National
    Committee for Mental Hygiene to Murray MacLaren, Minister of Pen-
    sions and National Health, 24 Nov. 1932.

38 PAC, DCH Minutes, 17th meeting, 19-21 June 1928, p. 3.

39 R. E. Wodehouse, *ibid.*, 33rd meeting, 2-3 Nov. 1936, p. 23.

40 PAC, RG 29, vol. 1062, file 502-1-1, part 1, letter from J. J.
    Heagerty of Department of Pensions and National Health to H. E.
    Spencer, M. P., 26 Apr. 1930.

41 J. T. Sproule, Commons, *Debates*, 1935, p. 185; J. P. Howden, *ibid.*,
    p. 1136.

42 Alexander M. Young, *ibid.*, 1938, pp. 1979-80.

43 Quoted by H. E. Spencer, *ibid.*, 1934, p. 500.

44 "Medical Relief," editorial, *CPHJ*, 25 (Apr. 1934), 187.

45 C. Howard Shillington, *The Road to Medicare in Canada* (Toronto:
    Del Graphics Pub., 1972), Preface.

46 PAC, DCH Minutes, 27th meeting, 16-18 Oct. 1933, p. 23.

47 For a sociological study of this problem, see Bernard R. Blishen,
    Doctors and Doctrines. The Ideology of Medical Care in Canada
    (Toronto: University of Toronto Press, 1969).

48 R. D. Morand, Commons, *Debates*, 1935, p. 182.

49   H. R. Fleming, Commons, *Debates*, 1938, pp. 1080-4; D. M. Suther-
     land, *ibid.*, 1935, p. 1137.

50   R. J. Manion, *ibid.*, 1919, p. 1182.

51   PAC, RG 29, vol. 858, file 20-C-33, part 1, letter from T. C.
     Routley of the CMA to Deputy Minister R. E. Wodehouse, 13 Feb.
     1940.

52   For a discussion of the hand the medical profession has in its own
     regulation in Canada and elsewhere see Malcolm G. Taylor, "The
     Role of the Medical Profession in the Formulation and Execution of
     Public Policy," *Canadian Journal of Economics and Political Science*,
     26 (Feb. 1960), 108-27; G. R. Weller, "Health Care and Medicare
     Policy in Ontario in *Issues in Canadian Public Policy*, ed. by Doern
     and Wilson; and Ivan Illich, *Limits to Medicine. Medical Nemesis:
     The Exploration of Health* (London: Marion Boyars, 1976).

53   Peebles, pp. 466-7. For a comparative study see James Sedley Cud-
     more, "A Comparative Study of Health Insurance and Public Medical
     Care Schemes in Germany, Great Britain, The United States of Ameri-
     ca, and Canada," unpublished Ph.D. dissertation, University of
     Toronto, 1951.

54   See Dickin McGinnis, chapter 6.

55   "Report of the Committee on Economics of the Canadian Medical As-
     sociation as presented at the Annual Meeting in Calgary June 18-
     22, 1934," *Canadian Medical Association Journal*, appended to the
     end of vol. 31.

56   See Canada, House of Commons, Special Committee on Social Security,
     Health Insurance, *Report of the Advisory Committee on Health In-
     surance* (Ottawa: King's Printer, 1943).

57   See *Ibid.* The files on health insurance in the papers of the De-
     partment of National Health and Welfare housed in the Public Ar-
     chives of Canada, are voluminous. See especially vols. 1058 to
     1144. Two detailed studies on the rise and fall of the health in-
     surance proposals have quite recently entered the literature. One
     is Robert S. Bothwell, "The Health of the Common People," in
     Mackenzie King, Widening the Debate, ed. John English and J. O.
     Stubbs (Toronto: Macmillan, 1977). He treats mostly the political
     aspects of the problem. The longer and more detailed work is the
     first chapter, "The 1945 Health Insurance Proposals: Policymaking
     for Post-War Canada," in Malcolm G. Taylor, *Health Insurance and
     Canadian Public Policy. The Seven Decisions that Created the
     Canadian Health Insurance System* (Montreal: McGill-Queen's Press,
     1978), pp. 1-68. See also Irving J. Goffman, "The Political His-
     tory of National Hospital Insurance in Canada," *Journal of Common-
     wealth Political Studies*, 3 (July 1965), 136-40.

58   H. M. Cassidy, *Social Security and Reconstruction in Canada* (Toron-
     to: Ryerson, 1943), p. 159. A. E. Grauer, *Public Health* (Ottawa:
     King's Printer, 1940), p. 74.

59   L. Richter, "The Effect of Health Insurance on the Demand for
     Health Services," *Canadian Journal of Economics and Political Sci-
     ence*, 10 (May 1944), 179-205.

60 Canada, Department of National Health and Welfare, *Social Security in Canada* (Ottawa: Information Canada, 1974), p. 3. Health Study Bureau, *Review of Canada's Health Needs and Health Insurance Proposals* (Toronto: the Board, 1945), pp. 11-22.

61 A. D. Watson, Chief Actuary, Department of Insurance. PAC, DCH Minutes, 41st meeting, 12-14 June 1941, p. 20-1.

62 H. E. MacDermot, "Health Insurance in Canada," *Queen's Quarterly*, 51 (Aug. 1944), 316.

63 D. L. Matters, "A Report on Health Insurance: 1919," *B. C. Studies*, 21 (Spring 1974), 28.

64 Daniel McIvor, Commons, *Debates*, 1938, p. 1070.

65 D. H. Williams, "Dominion Health Parade," *Canadian Affairs Pamphlets*, II (5) (Ottawa: King's Printer, 15 March 1945), 17.

66 MacDermot, "Health Insurance in Canada," p. 319.

67 Malcolm G. Taylor, *The Administration of Health Insurance in Canada* (Toronto: Oxford University Press, 1956), p. 212-13.

68 Taylor, "The Role of the Medical Profession in the Formulation and Execution of Public Policy," p. 114.

69 PAC, RG 29, vol. 1062, file 502-1-1, part 1, correspondence between the CMA and the Department, Dec. 1929 to Mar. 1930.

70 T. J. O'Neill, Commons, *Debates*, 1939 (1st session), pp. 1583-4.

71 PAC, RG 29, vol. 858, file 20-C-33, part 1, R. E. Wodehouse to T. H. Leggett, 15 June 1940.

72 *Ibid.*, vol. 613, file 339-5-2, J. J. Heagerty to R. E. Wodehouse, 28 Nov. 1939.

73 *Ibid.*, vol. 1107, file 504-1-2, part 1, correspondence between College and Department, Mar. to Dec. 1942.

74 For most of the correspondence between the Department and the CMA on health insurance, see PAC, RG 29, vol. 1111, file 304-2-4, part 1.

75 *Ibid.*, vol. 858, file 20-C-33, part 1, R. E. Wodehouse to T. C. Routley, 9 Sept. 1941.

76 *Canadian Medical Association Journal*, 46 (1942), 389. Quoted in H. E. MacDermot, "A Short History of Health Insurance in Canada," *Canadian Medical Association Journal*, 50 (May 1944), 452.

77 PAC, RG 29, vol. 1111, file 304-2-4, part 1, memo, J. J. Heagerty to Minister, 9 Apr. 1942. He did so.

78 R. S. Bothwell and J. R. English, "Pragmatic Physicians: Canadian Medicine and Health Care Insurance, 1910-1945," *University of Western Ontario Medical Journal*, 47 (Mar. 1976), 16.

79 Daniel McIvor, Commons, *Debates*, 1943, p. 153.

80 Taylor, "The Role of the Medical Profession," p. 119.

81 Prime Minister W. L. Mackenzie King admitted that "frankly I did not think the Treasury could stand it." Quoted in J. W. Pickersgill, *The Mackenzie King Record, Volume I, 1939-1944* (Toronto: University of Toronto Press, 1960), p. 636.

82 L. C. Marsh, *Social Security for Canada* (Ottawa: King's Printer, 1943), p. 28. Grauer, *Public Health*, p. 3.

83 Adelard Groulx, "A National Health Program, *CPHJ*, 24 (Jan. 1943), 13.

84 A. E. Grauer, *Public Assistance and Social Insurance* (Ottawa: Royal Commission on Dominion-Provincial Relations, 1940), p. 55.

85 J. J. Heagerty, PAC, DCH Minutes, 26th meeting, 13-15 June 1933, p. 25.

86 C. G. Power. See Commons, *Debates*, 1936, p. 2165-9.

87 Herbert A. Bruce, *ibid.*, 1940, p. 3823-4. Mackenzie King, *ibid.*, p. 4256. "Canada Needs a Department of Health," editorial, *CPHJ*, 35 (May 1944), 203-4.

88 See D. W. Gullett, *A History of Dentistry in Canada* (Toronto: University of Toronto Press for Canadian Dental Association, 1971), p. 207-12.

89 Name withheld. Personal interview, 8 June 1978.

MEDICINE AND THE STATE IN CANADA

ANNE CRICHTON

It is particularly appropriate to consider the relationship between organized medicine and the state at a time when a Royal Commission is considering how best to manage the tensions arising out of this relationship in Canada. As in other countries, the doctors of Canada play an important role in society, not only as diagnosticians and therapists, but also as gatekeepers, preserving social order through regulating deviant behavior and influencing individuals' willingness to conform to social norms. However, the behavior and role of doctors, as well as other professionals, are being questioned.

This paper offers an analysis of the response of organized medical care in Canada to government health care policies in terms of Terence J. Johnson's[1] paradigm, in which he suggests that professional groups may be viewed (1) as responding to patronage, (2) as collegial self-regulating associations, or (3) as groups whose behavior is mediated by the state or by the capitalist industrial system. While it seems that organized medicine in Canada may still be modelling itself on self-regulation, it may now be falling somewhere between the capitalist and state-mediated power situations.

I

The Professions in Society

Sociologists of all persuasions[2] agree that the function of the professions in a society is to provide social control--to act as gatekeepers for the society by guiding the citizens towards normative behavior. In consequence, it is important that professionals should reflect the "general will" of a society and should not be too far out of touch with its ideology and its dynamic, although lags are to be expected.

In the sixties, questions about the satisfactory functioning of the professions in the U.S.A. began to spill over the border into Canada. Were the doctors in Saskatchewan, who challenged the provincial government in 1962, firing the bullets for the American Medical Association[3] or for the Canadian medical profession itself? In either case, was the medical profession in Saskatchewan, at that time, in touch with Canadian aspirations? This professional group was a very privileged one--one of the few occupational groups which had been delegated monopoly powers in the nineteenth century. How did physicians use these powers? Were they behaving in a self-interested way? Were they responding adequately to the needs of society? How did they keep their own interests and those of society in balance?

The questions about American professions' lack of responsiveness to demands for social change grew more rapidly in the late sixties as the pressures for change in that society increased. Ivan Illich[4] challenged educators, physicians, and other occupational groups by developing the argument that this was "the age of the disabling professions" because professionals had created too great a dependency upon their services. Others, such as Thomas McKeown,[5] a Canadian working in England, demonstrated that the major contribution of the medical profession to increased health of populations had been in infection control, promotion of nutrition, and infant survival, and, now that these were well in hand in advanced technological societies, physicians were not improving life expectations to any great extent. Prolongation of life of reduced quality and iatrogenesis were quite as likely to be the results of physician intervention as "better health." On the other hand, a different sort of criticism of the professions in the U.S.A. was that they had a blinkered vision.[6] They were accused of concentrating on the one-to-one relationship of professional and client rather than looking at society as a whole and of failing to be disturbed by the maldistribution of professional services. Professionals were providing for the middle and upper classes but not for the poor, who were in more need of their help to cope with the stresses of modern life. There may seem to be some inconsistency in these two criticisms, but they came from two different radical perspectives.

That these criticisms were also expressed in Canada is quite clear. Illich and McKeown were invited to address Canadian audiences. A summary of Illich's criticisms concludes the collected papers of a seminar on professions and public policy[7] held in Toronto in 1976. McKeown strongly influenced the authors of *A New Perspective on the Health of Canadians*.[8]

A subcommittee of the Quebec (Castonguay)[9] investigation into provincial policy development in health and social affairs, set up to

examine the professions, accused them of failing to respond to the
needs of all the people of that province. Elsewhere,[10] provincial
governments established committees to examine whether the existing regulations were in need of revision in order to bring the professions
more in touch with the general social changes which had taken place in
the twentieth century. The Royal Commission on Health Services (1961-
64)[11] commissioned a special report on physician manpower supply and
distribution.[12]

II

Professional Roles

Since the professionals are gatekeepers, expected to exert control over behaviors of citizens, it is important that they should
understand and accept the current norms and future aspirations of society. This is by no means easy, for their social control function is
seldom openly discussed. Professional education is technical education. General education usually comes before or after specific medical, legal, or other programs of training. Attempts to introduce behavioral science courses into the designated professional stage of education have not been very successul because they seem to cut across
the concerns of the students at this point in their careers as they
move from being laymen to becoming one of the professional elite
through acquisition of technical skills.

Sociologists[13] have commented upon the way in which professionals
like to stress their technical abilities and to keep their other roles
ambiguous or discretionary, so that they have room for maneuver. And
the public goes along with this concern. The voices of sociologists
and economists who try to bring these other roles into the open are
seldom heard or, if heard, noticed and acted upon. Eliot Freidson,[14]
an American sociologist, has developed more thoroughly than others the
theme of increasing medical dominance in Western societies through the
greater amount of definition of abnormal behaviors as "sick," rather
than eccentric or criminal. Economists, such as R. G. Evans[15] or V. R.
Fuchs,[16] have been more concerned about professionals as resource allo-
cators--their wide range of discretionary activity in urgent, emergent,
and elective decision-making about diagnosis and treatment, and even
the necessity of return visits to the doctor's office.

III

Social Goals and Professional Goals

Policy analysts have made it clear that nations differ in their social ideologies,[17] so that while the Western democratic societies share some common aspirations, they have developed different ranges of values and organizational structures to realize them.[18] Thus, Canada differs from the other nations because of the particular way in which it has decided to pursue its value goals and to structure them into its national life.

M. P. Marchak[19] has explained Canadian ideologies as follows. There is a dominant liberal philosophy which is challenged by a more humanitarian approach. The (small l) liberalism is characterized by emphasis on relatively unrestricted entrepreneurial activity to develop national resources with the least possible government intervention, while the humanitarian challenge has been concerned with supporting those in need and the more equal distribution of resources to citizens. The responsibility for the major humanitarian measures seems to be moving from voluntary organizations to government sponsorship.[20]

An American political scientist, T. J. Lowi,[21] has argued that Western nations have moved through three phases of development. Initially, governments were concerned with *distribution* to supporters, later with *regulation*, and later still with *redistribution*. The aforementioned analyst of the professions, T. J. Johnson,[22] has quite independently suggested that these occupational groups may usefully be examined when under patronage, when they are self-regulating colleges, or when they are in a mediative situation controlled by the redistributive forces of (a) capitalism or (b) government.

As Johnson has pointed out, the professions would prefer to be in a collegiate control (or self-regulatory) position because in this relationship "the producer defines the needs of the consumer and the manner in which these needs are catered for." This is to be contrasted with patronage in which oligarchies, corporations, or community organizations impose upon producers their definitions of needs and the manner in which they are to be met. And then there is the situation in which "a third party mediates in the relationship between producer and consumer, defining both the needs and the manner in which these are met." The third party may be capitalism, "in which the capitalist entrepreneur intervenes in the direct relationship between the producer and

consumer in order to rationalize production and regulate markets. No
less significant, however, is state mediation. . .in which a powerful
centralized state intervenes in the relationship between producer and
consumer, initially to define what the needs are. . . ."[23]

How, then, do Canadian social goals and the goals of the medical
profession coincide? And at what stage of development are the Canadian
state and the Canadian medical profession, and are they in tune with
one another?

Like Johnson, I will start with self-regulation, then consider
patronage, then mediation, although Lowi has argued that distribution
comes before regulation and redistribution. Since the primary focus
of our attention is the practitioners, and then their context, let us
take the discussion in that order, for self-regulation focuses on internal professional processes, and patronage and redistribution focus
on external forces affecting the group.

A. Self-Regulation

In 1858, when the British medical profession managed to establish
the collegial self-regulating model, Canada was not even an independent
dominion, and so when the numbers of doctors became large enough to be
visible in Canada, this model was the current one used as the pattern
for development. In that year, the British government enacted regulations which provided for delegation of authority to a General Medical
Council manned by the profession. In return, the G.M.C. was to guarantee quality control over services, for now that medical learning was
demonstrably scientific, it was thought that no layman could judge competence.

It was in the 1860s, before Confederation, that medical groups began meeting in the centres of population in Canada. Under the British
North America Act (1867), health and welfare services were to be made a
provincial responsibility, with one or two program exceptions. In
practice, the provinces delegated their authority under regulations to
any group willing to provide these health and welfare services. Entrepreneurial physicians were spreading out across the North American con-
tinent, setting up in practice wherever they thought they could earn a
living, and forming collegial associations.[24] These were even less controlled than their British counterparts, for there was no discussion of
government appointments to their Councils. It must be recognized, of
course, that there was no other way in which provincial governments

could have regulated the professions at this time, for they had no administrative resources of their own.

Nor did the Canadian associations separate collegial business (i.e., quality control business) from association business (i.e., economic matters, such as fee scheduling), at least in the very early stages, though some did in the late nineteenth century and early twentieth century. (This lack of separation of powers could lead to difficulties later on, as it did in Saskatchewan in 1962.[25])

The professional associations' complete control over quality was modified to some extent in the early twentieth century. The concept of satisfactory quality control took a hard knock with the publication of the Flexner Report[26] to the Carnegie Foundation in 1910. This document criticized the poor standards of preparation in many U.S. and Canadian medical schools, and the institution of rigorous accreditation procedures followed. Another quality control mechanism was developed and became widely accepted around 1920, namely, voluntary hospital accreditation, which provided tests of continuing competence instead of entry tests alone. It was a Canadian, Malcolm McEachern, who went to the American College of Surgeons to bring in this extra-professional association control mechanism. He was greatly helped by getting support from the Catholic Hospital Association, which forced the municipal hospitals in Canada to follow their example.[27] But today there is still no similar control over office practice.

Economic control was purely an internal matter to the associations at this stage. Rules were devised to regulate advertising, fee-splitting, and other referral practices so that "professional ethics" would be observed. (Later, after the introduction of Medicare, the profession developed economic monitoring through comparison of practice profiles of members, in order to prevent government monitoring from becoming the only control.)

The activities of the medical profession regarding health planning and continuing education must be commended. In comparison with other professional groups, they have provided an excellent example.

B. Patronage in the Health Services

I would now like to consider this concept in three steps:

1. Institutions or Doctors' Workshops. As B. Abel-Smith[28] has pointed out, it is important to examine the basic historical reasons for establishing health services in a country. In Britain and

Australia, hospitals began as asylums for the poor and developed into
medical teaching centres, while in the U.S.A., doctors generally directed their services towards the middle classes. When hospitals were
built, they were of many different kinds: teaching and nonteaching, in
profit and nonprofit settings, missionary, municipal, doctor-owned,
prepaid plan-owned, etc., but the major emphasis was on profit-making
hospitals.

The model chosen for the development of health service institutions in Canada was a modified American plan, not the British model,
and in this endeavor local communities were actively engaged in working
for and with the doctors to establish hospitals as their workshops.
The Hospital Boards limited their activities to management of resources,
not programs of care, which were left to the doctors to initiate. G.
Harvey Agnew[29] has explained how Canada came late to the hospital building game. Up to about 1920, Canadians were not particularly willing to
trust hospitals, and most medical care was given in the home. When
hospitals were built, they were usually missionary or non-profit community projects.

A few Canadian hospitals in the larger cities had charity wards,
but in general across the country it was not practical to segregate the
poor from the rest of the patients. Canadian doctors seem to have accepted that general hospitals should be provided by nonprofit societies.
They seem to have recognized that having access to these workshops gave
them many hidden subsidies which could be exploited if they were good
managers[30] and that there was not the population base for medical entrepreneurial activity, except in chronic care hospital provision. The
Canadian health care industry thus seems to have been small and underdeveloped before 1949 when the federal government began to put money
into the health care system.

In 1949 the federal government introduced the first two stages of
the national insurance programs--public and mental health grants and
the hospital construction program. In the eyes of the federal government this was a redistributive program, but in the eyes of others at
lower levels of government, it seems to have been viewed as an extension of earlier patronage activities.

The hospital construction program was to have been based on written
provincial redistribution plans, but when these were produced, they were
not carried out. It took provincial governments until the late sixties
to develop mechanisms of control, for they had no strong administrators
who could manage the political pressures from municipalities.

    2. <u>The Flow of Patients and Organization of Services</u>. A second
form of patronage is not concerned with the distribution of construction contracts, but with the flow of patients through the system and
the organization of categories and programs of service.

    In Canada, the medical profession has managed to avoid being
placed under the more obvious aspects of service patronage, except for
a few occupational health officers who have chosen to work for corporations. The later development of hospitals (mainly after 1949) meant
that the British struggles[31] about subscriber patronage were over, and
that doctors had long won the battle for control over admitting patients and peers.[32] Nevertheless Canadian doctors appear to have a
strong fear of being put into the position of reporting back to community organizations. The medical profession's reaction to the concept of
Community Health Centres[33] was strongly hostile, no doubt in large part
for this reason. Recent challenges in hospital settings--the abortion
issue particularly--have not only divided local communities but pose
new problems of board-physician relationships[34] because hospital boards
are seeking new power to interfere in program development.

    The strength of physicians' hostility to any control by community
and consumer groups, whether in clinics, hospitals, or through government plans, is interesting in a country where service patronage of physicians really has not existed (the exception being contract doctoring
in company towns). It can best be explained by the reaction of
British immigrant physicians, refugees from the National Health Service, who brought with them a mythology about the struggles of their
predecessors in the nineteenth century to free themselves from contract
doctoring, ministering to those patients chosen by subscribers to voluntary hospitals, or working for local authorities (which was the major
point of issue in 1911 when National Health Insurance was introduced).[35]

    3. <u>Physicians and Big Business</u>. It would appear, then, that Cana-
dian physicians have managed to resist patronage, at least at one level,
for very few of them are working directly for corporations or other employers who give the orders. Nevertheless, there is a deeper criticism
of physicians developed by Marxists and other radicals. McKinlay[36] has
called physicians "the willing tools of big business" in the U.S., and
Navarro[37] has documented their gatekeeping activities on behalf of international capitalism. The big business in the U.S. is, of course,
medical technology and the hospitals which contain it. While there are
strong pressures in Canada to keep up with the latest developments in
medical equipment and supplies, there has been some resistance to

international capitalism. The federal government (and later some provincial governments) took steps to regulate the pharmaceutical industry
when it fell under complete American control in the early sixties. R.
W. Lang had documented the struggle of the Ottawa civil servants working together with a Senate Committee to make public the issues and to
develop some counteraction. Lang's report showed that the Canadian
Medical Association provided strong support to the case of the pharmaceutical industry and against the case of the federal government in the
inquiries[38] which dragged on through the sixties.

In the light of Lang's arguments, it is necessary to ask whether
the medical profession, which creates an image of humanitarianism, is
not in fact at the right-wing extreme of Marchak's schema of liberalism,
that is, willing to be patronized by "big business" so that it can profit by "distribution" and "self-regulation" while the *federal* government
has moved to take up the challenging humanitarian "redistribution" position.

However, both dominant and challenging ideologies in Canada accept
the need for a disciplined work force geared to production. The humani-
tarians are just more concerned about picking up the pieces. Yet there
are new ideological challenges beginning to emerge--as exemplified by
the ten-year legacy of the flower children who did not want to devote
their lives to work--but they have been tamed by recession. Now working
people themselves are questioning the healthfulness of their environments
more fiercely than ever before. We can expect to see much more of their
challenge to big business and its capabilities for control.

C. Mediation

Lowi's third stage, redistribution of services, became an issue in
the thirties, when the great depression affected the country, when cash
became short and barter common. Agnew[39] described the plight of Canadian hospitals which could not raise money within their communities, and
all service providers had difficulties in getting debts paid. The provincial governments themselves sought financial relief in constitutional
revision, and the Rowell-Sirois Commission was set up to investigate
federal-provincial relationships.[40] At the local level, one province,
Saskatchewan, devised a municipal doctor scheme[41] whereby physicians
were paid salaries by local communities so that they would not leave
these areas which had become accustomed to rely on professional help,
though elsewhere in Canada the free market prevailed.

As the Rowell-Sirois Committee reported in 1940, constitutional
revisions were deferred because of the war. However, in 1943, influenced by investigations of New Deal policies in America and postwar
reconstruction plans for Britain, the federal government set up two
committees to investigate the social security of Canadians--the Marsh
Committee[42] with a broad general mandate, and the Heagerty Committee[43]
with instructions to examine national health insurance. The medical
profession was closely involved in the latter and agreed to support
the development of a national health insurance program, for prepayment
schemes had not, at that time, made much headway in Canada[44] and, where
they had been introduced, the insured had chosen hospital care options
rather than medical care schemes. So the proposed national insurance
scheme promised much greater economic security than the profession had
had before.

The long-drawn-out series of bargaining sessions between federal
and provincial governments, first about methods of financing the new
social security programs while maintaining the constitutional rights of
the provinces, and then about priorities in programming, are succinctly
described in the Canada Year Books.[45] The Year Books also describe the
changes in the Canadian social structure over this thirty-five-year
postwar period--the growth in population from 11 to 22 million and its
continuing redistribution from rural into urban areas. As well, the
economic development of the country is chronicled--its transformation
from a poor, depressed agricultural country in the thirties to one of
the richest nations in the world in the seventies.

While the interests of the medical profession coincided with those
of the federal government in the forties, they began to drift apart
through the fifties and the commitment to redistribution made in the
forties began to seem less appealing to them as the years wore on. Was
this new wealth not the result of private enterprise--of individual
initiatives? Had collectivism not gone far enough in providing traditional public health services and financing general hospitals with the
promise (still to be implemented in 1965) of revised pension schemes
yet to come? Doctors had set up their own nonprofit fee prepayment
schemes and were not anxious to have government programs instead.[46] By
the early sixties, it was felt to be important to test the general will
about further action on national health insurance and a Royal Commission[47] was set up to inquire into the health needs of Canadians. It
was after this committee was appointed that the Saskatchewan government

introduced a Medical Care program in 1962 and faced a strike, by the
majority of the provincial medical profession, which lasted 23 days.[48]
Nevertheless, the Hall Commission reported in 1964 in favor of introducing a federal Medical Care scheme and this plan was enacted in 1966.

It seems that the agreement of the Canadian medical professional
groups to go along with this scheme rested upon ambiguities. Were the
physicians to become subsidized entrepreneurs or contractors to governments? The Saskatoon Agreement which ended the strike of 1962 was concerned with several different issues:

> The government wanted a plan providing universal
> coverage, known patient liability, and unified
> administration. The profession regarded these
> principles as false principles harmful to both
> patients and doctors. In general the settlement
> provided a face-saving device....It is ironical
> that Lord Taylor, a neuropsychiatrist, helped to
> provide a solution to the impasse that served to
> delude both the profession and the public.[49]

In order to reach agreement, important issues were left ambiguous and
unclarified, so that the doctors could resume work and the government
could meet its promises. These were still left ambiguous when the
federal scheme was introduced. Particularly important was the issue:
"Were the doctors to regard themselves as subsidized entrepreneurs or
in contract with the government if they took Medicare money?" It was
put in a slightly different way by D. Geekie of the Canadian Medical
Association in a recent statement:

> CMA feels that without the right to bill patients,
> Medicare becomes in effect a state medical scheme
> where the doctor becomes an employee and responsi-
> ble to the state rather than responsible to and an
> advocate for the patient.[50]

After the introduction of government-subsidized medical care negotiations about day-to-day matters between professional associations
and provincial governments went relatively smoothly for a number of
years. Increases in fee schedules, set by the professional associations, had been brought in just before the federal/provincial Medicare
program was introduced into most provinces. As well, bad debts were
eliminated and the volume of services by individual physicians frequently rose. R. G. Evans[51] has shown how the immediate result was a rise
in incomes. However, by 1977 when the federal/provincial funding
agreements were renegotiated, the physicians were already beginning to
feel left behind in the professional race. Overheads were rising and
so they felt poorer in absolute terms and, as well, their relative income position appeared to have declined. They no longer perceived

themselves to be clearly ahead of all other occupational groups in
earning incomes. In several provinces they began to bill their patients for additional amounts beyond those paid from government funds.
An attempt by the Liberal federal Minister of Health to deal with this
directly vis-à-vis the Province of Ontario in May 1979[52] was cut short
by a federal election. The new Conservative government invited Mr.
Justice Emmett Hall to re-examine health care issues and report back.
This he was scheduled to do in the fall of 1980, despite a further
change in government.[53]

It will be recognized that Canadian governments have become involved in mediation at a time when questions are being worked through
about the extent of the federal responsibility for providing "welfare
state" services. Ideologies are not clear-cut but vary right across
the country. And the issues of structuring mediative control are complex. First, there is the issue of using market forces versus government or bureaucratic forces as the mediating agent. Where does Canada
stand in this? A discussion on the professions and public policy held
in Toronto in 1976 had advocates for both approaches.[54] Second, there
is the issue of who is to define health and sickness. In the capitalist model this is delegated to the doctors, but there are questions
about whether they follow the directions of "big business" pushing high
technology and/or tranquilizers.

Wildavsky[55] has pointed out that there tends to be a displacement
of health objectives by citizens. Because good health is an elusive
goal, citizens ask for health care, and because good health care cannot
easily be judged, access to health care has been substituted for health
itself. John Evans[56] makes clear that some access is important and
worthwhile, but questions just how much is necessary.

A large step forward in the Canadian state mediative situation was
taken when the Lalonde Working Document was given such an enthusiastic
reception. *A New Perspective on the Health of Canadians* has removed
"health" from the total control of physicians by emphasizing personal
responsibility for lifestyles and environment, as well as high risk.[57]
However, the definition of "sickness" still remains a medical matter,
and in Canada, as in those other Western countries which feel strongly
about the Protestant ethic, there has been a tendency to stigmatize
anyone dropping out of society's normal patterns unless they are designated "sick." Great efforts have been made by European welfare state
societies to change this, to allow citizens to drop out for other

reasons and get social work or other supports as well as or instead of
medical care. Canada is uncertain whether to allow this to happen, because this social policy denies the concepts of individual responsibility and free enterprise, and of personal control over life decisions.
A study of home care policies, province by province, has shown that
Quebec, Saskatchewan, and Manitoba are more willing to recognize non-
medical dropouts than are the other provinces.[58]

Third, there is the issue of the allocation of resources in the
redistribution of wealth or rationing of scarce services. As we have
seen, the Saskatchewan doctors regarded principles of universality,
known patient liability, and universal administration as "false principles"--thus illustrating that values are controversial. Structural-
ly, financial resources can be relatively easily controlled by nonpro-
fessionals, but the allocation of service resources is linked to clinical judgments and how far professional discretion is allowed to extend.
Once the issue of clinical judgment is raised, the argument is closed
off, except for the area surrounding the judgments, so discussion of
the topic becomes displaced onto the organization of the settings in
which clinical judgments take place, such as the availability of hospital beds by area or by specialty.

In a study of rationing of social services in Britain, K. Judge[59]
discussed the distinction between financial rationing and service
rationing, the former being undertaken by politicians and bureaucrats,
the latter to some extent by bureaucrats but mainly by professionals.
The mediative state must be concerned about both kinds of rationing because they are the methods of controlling what services are to be delivered. While financial rationing is open to discussion of principles
(such as universality versus selectivity), service rationing is often
idiosyncratic, expedient, and inequitable. R. A. Parker[60] classified
service rationing into three activities--restrictive (explicit or implied deterrence--the uses of eligibility criteria, charges, or delay),
dilutant (reduction of services to individual clients), and early ter-
mination of service. These categories give some indication of its dis-
criminatory uses and possible abuses. When there are real differences
in values between professionals and governments, service rationing may
be used to defy governments which are supposed to express "the general
will" of citizens.

I believe that the mediative state requires a strong bureaucracy
to try to bring financial and service rationing into relationship with

each other. This is what seems to be developing in Canada--and this is
what the Saskatchewan doctors were afraid of. It is noticeable that in
the last decade the provincial health (and other civil service) departments are becoming much stronger, manned by professionally-trained administrators rather than professionals turned administrator or upgraded
clerks. However, the seniors among these professional administrators
are expected to have served their time in the field so that they can
bring specific knowledge to the solution of problems--that is, they also know how service rationing works, as well as understanding financial
rationing.

Canada has a tradition of using a wide range of formal and informal committees to resolve or defer conflicts rather than allowing open
confrontation between polarized groups, which might easily happen to
governments and professions, as in Australia. Thus, it is to be expected that the new bureaucrats would use these buffering mechanisms in
their struggles for control over the health services. The use of Hall
as the Commissioner of the Health Services Review '79 is one example of
this. In British Columbia, which is the only province I know well, the
government is working closely with the B.C. Hospital Association--a
consortium of trustees and their administrators--to develop a new method of funding hospitals[61] and a different way of classifying their activities.[62] Regional districts in B.C. were set up in 1966 to buffer
the government against municipal demands for hospital capital funding.
The activities of the regional advisory committees in Ontario and Quebec, which deal not only with capital but operational spending, are
being watched by the B.C. government with interest, for it is recognized that hospitals cannot be considered separately from other health
service provision. As well, grassroots consumers organized into regional advisory groups could become important allies for the bureaucrats in determining priorities in spending. As yet, however, Quebec's
experience has been that regional, district, and local health centre
management groups soon revert to letting themselves become dominated by
professionals rather than consumers, despite all efforts to increase
consumer involvement.[63]

Less obliquely and more in a spirit of confrontation, in the early
seventies several provincial governments decided to set up committees
of inquiry into the professions. In Quebec,[64] this activity resulted
in the establishment of an Office of the Professions which now regu-
lates the activities of 38 professional groups. In Ontario, a

Committee on the Healing Arts examined professional manpower and its
deployment; in Alberta, a Special Committee of the Legislature considered professional organization; in Manitoba and Saskatchewan citizens'
rights vis-à-vis professionals were examined. The Ontario Medical Association itself initiated an investigation[65] in response to consumer
concerns and recommended the appointment of lay representatives to the
O.M.A. Council. Some might regard this as a pre-emptive procedure before governments got into the act of stiffening regulations, for laymen
invited to attend professional association councils can easily be dominated.

V

Conclusions

Canada has not yet decided how best to handle the management of
the professions in the eighties. The provinces which have had the
greatest open controversies between physicians and governments have
been:

(a) Saskatchewan, 1962, upon the introduction of Medicare legislation and the community clinics;[66]

(b) Quebec, 1970, when the specialists struck against the introduction of Medicare.[67] Many have since left the province just as
many Saskatchewan doctors left after their strike. The Centres
locales de Service Communautaire issue has also been current;[68]

(c) Manitoba, 1972, when the medical profession reacted strongly
to the government White Paper on the organization of services[69]
but worked out a satisfactory relationship; and

(d) Ontario and Alberta, 1979, on the issue of extra billing beyond Medical Care payments--an issue referred to the Hall Commission.

In these controversies there have been value issues and structural
issues. T. R. Marmor,[70] an American political scientist, has suggested that it is important to determine the "frame of inference" for analyzing the handling of policy issues, and points out that there can be
a series of different ways of conceptualizing problems. R. R. Alford,[71]
similarly, has demonstrated that groups who are using these different
frames of inference may never resolve their differences, that they may
go on meeting for years to plan health services without moving forward
to satisfactory resolutions. Canadians must recognize that this is a

distinct possibility. But at least the Canadian medical profession and
governments are talking, like the British and unlike the Americans and
Australians.

It is good to think that the Hall Commission is trying to do some
sorting for us, to clarify what "the general will" of Canadians is at
the present time. However, it will then be necessary to see whether
the doctors will be willing to respond to this federal expression of
opinion. Bernard Blishen,[72] the research director of the previous Hall
Commission, made a study of the medical profession's ideologies in 1962
and concluded that they were defensive and maladaptive to change. Yet,
there has been a considerable measure of change since then, so there
seems to be some hope for the future. However, accommodation between
negotiating groups will not come quickly, and oblique approaches would
seem to offer the best hopes for achieving them.

It seems to be agreed that the regulation of the professions is
overdue for change. However, it is not clear how best to make change.
There are different views reflecting different ideological stances from
"let them be controlled by capitalist mediation" (i.e., open up the professional monopolies to increase competition) to "let them be controlled
by state mediation" (i.e., stronger bureaucratic control). In 1976, a
symposium on *The Professions and Public Policy*[73] brought together the
views of prominent Canadian academics and civil servants on a series of
topics: professional regulation, professional education and regulation
of continuing competence, professional manpower and the use of parapro-
fessionals, access to professional services, and a discussion of employed professionals. This was where the differences in view emerged.

It seems likely that, as the century wears on, the physicians will
be brought into a mixture of mediative models of capitalist competitive
and state bureaucratic controls. Financial rationing procedures are
rapidly being streamlined, and service rationing procedures are being
questioned more and more as governments and consumers are reconsidering
the fundamental issues in health policy. As Fuchs puts it, "Who shall
live?"[74] and as others ask, "What about the quality of life of those who
are kept alive?" There will be many discussions of "medical ethics" in
this new interpretation relating to resource allocation in the years to
come.[75]

In the sixties, the search for Canadian identity was frequently
discussed. In the eighties, we are concerned lest the country should
fall apart, for it is a pluralist multicultural society with many rifts.
Perhaps we should not be surprised that the medical profession finds it

difficult to know what the norms are that they should seek to promote,
other than their own personal values. What we must admire is their organization in groups thinking about structures, whether as health planners or collective bargainers. Until other groups emerge which can
present alternatives with the same power, we must expect their views to
be dominant in our health policy-making.

NOTES

1 Terence J. Johnson, *Professions and Power* (London: Macmillan, 1972).

2 C. K. Watkins, *Social Control* (London: Longman, 1975); T. Parsons,
   The Social System (London: Tavistock, 1952); V. Navarro, "Social
   Class, Political Power and the State and Their Implications in
   Medicine," *Social Science and Medicine*, 10 (1976), 437-457.

3 *Financial Post*, July 14, 1962. Editorial: "Human Rights Mainly
   Duties," cited in R. F. Badgley and S. Wolfe, *Doctor's Strike*
   (Toronto: Macmillan, 1967), p. 69.

4 I. D. Illich, *Medical Nemesis* (London: Calder and Boyars, 1975).

5 T. J. McKeown, "The Determinants of Human Health: Behavior, Envir-
   onment, and Therapy," in W. C. Gibson, ed. *Health Care Teaching and
   Research* (Vancouver: U.B.C. Alumni Association and The Faculty of
   Medicine, 1975), pp. 58-77.

6 M. Rein, *Social Policy* (New York: Random House, 1970).

7 P. Slayton, and M. Trebilcock, eds., *The Professions and Public
   Policy* (Toronto: Toronto University Press, 1978).

8 Canada, Department of National Health and Welfare, *A New Perspective
   on the Health of Canadians* (Ottawa: Information Canada, 1974
   [Lalonde]).

9 Quebec, *The Professions and Society*, Report of the Commission of Inquiry into Health and Social Welfare, VII, Tome 1, Part 5 (Quebec:
   Government of Quebec, 1970).

10 Alberta, Reports of the Special Committee of the Legislative Assembly of Alberta on Professions and Occupations (Edmonton: Government
   Printer, I Apr. and II Dec., 1973); Ontario, Reports of the Committee on the Healing Arts (Toronto: Queen's Printer, 1970); Manitoba,
   Government evaluation of public policy towards the professions (in
   progress); Saskatchewan, Evaluation of citizens' rights to health
   care (in progress).

11 Canada, Report of the Royal Commission on Health Services (Ottawa:
   Queen's Printer, 1964 [Hall]).

12 S. Judek, *Medical Manpower in Canada*, Royal Commission on Health
   Services (Ottawa: Queen's Printer, 1964).

13 J. Jamous and B. Pelloille, "Professions or Self-Perpetuating Sys-
   tems? Changes in the French University Hospital System," in J. A.
   Jackson, ed., *Professions and Professionalization* (London: Cambridge
   University Press, 1970).

14 E. Freidson, *The Profession of Medicine* (New York: Dodd Mead, 1970).

15 R. G. Evans, "Economic Perspective," in S. Andreopoulos, ed., *National Health Insurance: Can the U.S. Learn from Canada?* (New York: Wiley and Sons, 1975).

16 V. R. Fuchs, *Who Shall Live?* (New York: Basic Books, 1974).

17 E.g., R. M. Titmuss, *Social Policy* (London: George Allen and Unwin, 1974).

18 R. M. Titmuss, *The Gift Relationship* (London: George Allen and Unwin, 1971).

19 M. P. Marchak, *Ideological Perspectives on Canada* (Toronto: McGraw Hill-Ryerson, 1975).

20 N. Carter, *Trends in Voluntary Support for NonGovernmental Social Service Agencies* (Ottawa: Canadian Council on Social Development, 1974).

21 T. J. Lowi, "American Business, Public Policy, Case-Studies and Political Theory," *World Politics*, 16 (1964), 677-715.

22 T. J. Johnson, *Professions and Power*.

23 *Ibid.*, pp. 45-46.

24 Archives of provincial colleges; G. W. Grove, *Organized Medicine in Ontario*, Report to the Committee on the Healing Arts (Toronto: Queen's Printer, 1970).

25 R.F. Badgley and S. Wolfe, *Doctors' Strike* (Toronto: MacMillan, 1967).

26 Abram Flexner, *Report on American Colleges* (New York: Carnegie Foundation, 1910).

27 G. Harvey Agnew, *Canadian Hospitals 1920-70* (Toronto: University of Toronto Press, 1974).

28 B. Abel-Smith, "The History of Medical Care," in E. W. Martin, ed., *Comparative Development in Social Welfare* (London: George Allen and Unwin, 1972), pp. 219-39. B. Abel-Smith, *The Hospitals 1800-1948* (London: Heinemann, 1964); K. S. Inglis, *Hospital and Community: A History of the Royal Melbourne Hospital* (Carlton: Melbourne University Press, 1958).

29 G. H. Agnew, *Canadian Hospitals 1920-70*.

30 A. O. J. Crichton, and D. O. Anderson, *Group Practice in the System* (Vancouver: University of British Columbia, 1973).

31 B. Abel-Smith, *The Hospitals 1800-1948*.

32 Some questions were raised, however, about admission to hospital privileges in Canadian hospitals in 1963 and 1972 when the behavior of peers was investigated viz: Saskatchewan, Commission of Inquiry into Hospital Privileges (Regina: Queen's Printer, 1963); Ontario, Committee of Inquiry into Hospital Privileges in Ontario (Toronto: Ministry of Health, 1972).

33 Canada, Department of National Health and Welfare, *The Community Health Centre* (Ottawa: Information Canada, 1972 and 1973), 3 vols. (Hastings).

34 J. Borthwick, "Case Study on the Polarization of a Board" (Vancouver: University of British Columbia, Department of Health Care and Epidemiology, 1980 [mimeo]).

35 R. Stevens, *Medical Practice in Modern England: The Impact of Specialization and State Medicine* (New Haven: Yale University Press, 1966).

36 J. B. McKinlay, "The Business of Good Doctoring or Doctoring as Good Business: Reflections on Freidson's Views of the Medical Game," *International Journal of Health Services*, 7, No. 3 (1977), 459-83.

37 V. Navarro, "Social Class, Political Power and the State and Their Implications in Medicine," *loc. cit.* 437-457.

38 R. W. Lang, *The Politics of Drugs* (Lexington, Mass.: Saxon House, 1974).

39 Agnew, *Canadian Hospitals 1920-70*.

40 Canada, Royal Commission on Dominion-Provincial Relations (Ottawa: King's Printer, 1940).

41 Badgley and Wolfe, *Doctors' Strike*, pp. 7-10.

42 Canada, *Social Security for Canada*, Report of the Advisory Committee on Reconstruction (Ottawa: King's Printer, 1943 [Marsh]).

43 Canada, *Health Insurance*, Report of the Advisory Committee on Health Insurance (Ottawa: King's Printer, 1943 [Heagerty]).

44 Agnew, *Canadian Hospitals 1920-70*.

45 *Canada Year Book, 1978-9* (Ottawa: Information Canada, 1979).

46 C. H. Shillington, *The Road to Medicare* (Toronto: DelGraphics, 1972).

47 Canada, Report of the Royal Commission on Health Services, pp. 723-740.

48 Badgley and Wolfe, *Doctors' Strike*.

49 *Ibid.*, p. 97.

50 D. Geekie, "Canadian Medical Association," in *University Affairs* (May, 1980), 5.

51 R. G. Evans, "Economic Perspective."

52 Canadian Newsfacts, 1979. *Bégin Warns Ontario on Medicare*, p. 2135.

53 Canada, *Health Services Review '79* (in progress).

54 P. Slayton and M. Trebilcock, eds., *The Professions and Public Policy*.

55 A. Wildavsky, "Doing Better and Feeling Worse," in J. H. Knowles, ed., *Doing Better and Feeling Worse* (New York: Norton & Co., 1977).

56 J. R. Evans, "Worldwide Health: Quality, Availability, Resources and Opportunities for International Collaboration," *Health Management Forum*, 1, No. 1 (Spring 1980), 6-19.

57 Canada, Department of National Health and Welfare, *A New Perspective on the Health of Canadians*, p. 18.

58 A. Crichton, *A Review of Community Health Care Services, 1980*, unpublished paper for the Health Services Review '79 (Vancouver: University of British Columbia, 1980).

59 K. Judge, *Rationing Social Services* (London: Heinemann, 1978).

60 R. A. Parker, "Social Administration and Scarcity," *Social Work*, 24 No. 2 (April 1967), 9-14.

61 British Columbia, Ministry of Health, Hospital Funding Study, *Evaluation and Recommendations*, vol. 1 (Victoria: Ministry of Health, 1979 [Ernst and Whinney]).

62 British Columbia, *Hospital Role Study*, *Phase 1* (Victoria: Ministry of Health, August 1979 [Pallan and Layton]).

63 M. Brunet and A. Vinet, *Les Professions: Un obstacle au changement social?* (Quebec: University of Laval, 1978 [mimeo]).

64 Quebec, *L'evolution du professionalisme au Québec*. Office des Professions du Quebec, September 1976.

65 E. A. Pickering, *Report of the Special Study regarding the Medical Profession in Ontario* (Toronto: Ontario Medical Association, 1973).

66 Badgley and Wolfe, *Doctors' Strike*.

67 M. G. Taylor, "Quebec Medicare: Problem Formulation in Conflict and Crisis," *Canadian Public Administration*, 15 (Summer 1972), 211-50.

68 G. Desrosiers, "The Introduction of a Network of Local Community Health Centres: 4 Years of Experience," *Canadian Journal of Public Health*, 69 (Jan.-Feb. 1978), 9.

69 Manitoba. Cabinet Committee on Health, Education and Social Policy, *White Paper on Health Policy* (Winnipeg: Government of Manitoba, 1972).

70 T. R. Marmor, *The Politics of Medicare* (Chicago: Aldine, 1973).

71 R. R. Alford, *Health Care Politics* (Chicago: University of Chicago Press, 1975).

72 B. Blishen, *Doctors and Doctrines* (Toronto: University of Toronto Press, 1969).

73 P. Slayton and M. Trebilcock, eds., *The Professions and Public Policy*.

74 V. R. Fuchs, *Who Shall Live?*

75 G. McLachlan, ed., *Patient, Doctor, Society* (London: Oxford University Press, 1972). S. J. Reiser, A. J. Dyck, and W. J. Curran, *Ethics in Medicine* (Cambridge, Mass.: M.I.T. Press).

COMMENTS ON THE PAPERS OF MCGINNIS AND CRICHTON

MALCOLM C. BROWN

At the outset I might mention that I found the paper of Dr. McGinnis relatively difficult to assess. The basic problem was that it involves not just one topic but three, and sometimes the topics are merged in a rather confusing way by fairly peculiar and implicit definitions of certain terms. As the title of the paper implies, it considers certain public health issues. But in addition it deals extensively with the political-economic behavior of the medical profession, both separately and in interaction with government bureaucracies. Finally, it considers certain dimensions of the evolution of Canada's curative care system, from one of private finance to one of "socialized" medicine.

The most obvious example of a peculiar definition of terms relates to the concept of public health. As I read the paper, public health is considered to be any kind of health activity which is publicly financed. This is not a conventional definition, and in my view not a particularly useful one. In economics, a public good, in contrast to a private good, is one where the exclusion principle does not hold. The exclusion principle, when applied to a commodity or service, simply means that the individual who consumes it receives all the utility which the good has. In effect, his consumption automatically means that others are excluded from enjoying the same output. A typical private good might be an ice cream, where the person who eats it is assumed to receive most, if not all, of the pleasure from the consumption. In contrast, a light-house beacon is often considered to be a good example of a public good, because if the light is turned on for one ship, all ships in the vicinity can benefit from it. In effect, a public good is one where collective consumption occurs because of the nature of the good, and consequently collective or public financing is necessary if one is to get an optimal amount of it.

Health professionals tend to think of public health as preventive health, in contrast to curative care. Sanitation and sewage programs, vaccination and inoculation programs, and environmental control programs are all normally included in the list of public health goods. It is of interest that this list primarily involves goods which a community can consume more efficiently than can an individual. In other words, it includes what economists would think of as public goods.

It was in the context of this kind of definition that I was originally extremely curious to see what Dr. McGinnis would find to say about public health programs during 1919-1945. The heyday of public health was really prior to this period, encompassing the years from 1865 to 1921.[1] Starting with Pasteur's work in the 1860s, and expanded by the efforts of others throughout the rest of the century, man learned much about how infectious diseases are transmitted, but almost nothing about how to arrest them in process. This development set the stage for substantial improvements and expansions in public health programs during the first two decades of the twentieth century. The setting up of public health departments was really just icing on the cake, done when all of the available scientific knowledge had been acted upon.

If 1900 to 1921 represents the heyday of public health, 1921 to 1966 represents the heyday of private-enterprise, curative-care medicine. The discovery of insulin in 1921, and the further discoveries of the sulphonamides and penicillin in the late 1930s and early 1940s gave medical practitioners a solid technological base with which they could impress patients with their worth. This base was exploited with considerable skill to justify high incomes for doctors.

In this context, it must be recalled that since the beginning of modern medicine (1865), doctors have always supported government policies involving care for the poor and the indigent. People forget that capitation was introduced in Britain in 1911 at the medical profession's request, to finance care which had originally been charity work. What the profession has always been opposed to is policies restricting their power to price patients who can pay.

The above backdrop is necessary to understand Canadian developments during the 1920s and 1930s. Since health departments were created after the major public health developments had occurred, their role in this area was relegated to the relatively minor function of co-ordinating programs. Given bureaucratic behavior, it was natural that they should attempt to expand their horizons. What better area for doing this than social welfare, where many of the policies would not only alleviate poverty but also improve health in ways favored by the medical profession. As Dr. McGinnis points out, the medical men

at the helm of most health departments found this course of action ir-
resistible.

The Great Depression, of course, did constitute a major problem
for the medical profession, as it did for most groups. But it did not
significantly change their views on economic policy. They still favored government finance of medical care for those who could not afford
to pay. However, under the circumstances, this began to look very much
like a program of national health insurance. If one reads carefully
the Saskatchewan Medical Association's endorsement of national health
insurance during the 1930s, it is clear that it did so only if the profession retained control over prices. Of course, given the relationship between the profession and health departments, it was natural for
the profession to believe that this control was not only possible but
likely.

The reason private-enterprise, curative-care medicine came to an
end was that physicians were just a little too successful in convincing
society of the worth of their product. Most people came around to the
view that more curative care meant better health. The problem was how
to achieve the objective. Providing more services at more affordable
prices was possible through either a more competitive supply of physicians or socialized medicine, but both options were resisted by the
profession.

In historical terms, the Canadian medical profession has been extraordinarily successful in resisting change. But change is inevitable. In this case, when change did occur, it involved public finance
rather than competition. This was so because most people accepted the
view of the medical profession that treatment is "complicated by the
availability of complex and expensive forms of technology that not only
require expertise to make them effective but can render lethal results
in the hands of the untrained."[2]

When did the golden age of private enterprise medicine end? I
have chosen 1966 with the passing of the Federal *Medical Care Act*.
However, the dating is always somewhat arbitrary, and other choices are
possible. The rationale of Dr. McGinnis's choice of 1945 would, I
would guess, be based on the fact that the first national proposal for
comprehensive public insurance was brought forward in that year. While
the proposal was unsuccessful, it could be argued that it represented
the beginning of the end.

Professor Crichton's objective of analyzing the "interaction of medical professional groups with federal and provincial governments" is both a timely and an important one. I only wish that she had pursued this task somewhat more vigorously in her paper. Instead she digresses to consider such matters as (1) social ideologies in Canada, (2) the medical profession's reaction to patronage, (3) the history of health finance, and (4) the disillusionment of academics with the effectiveness of curative care in the 1970s. Doubtless all of these matters relate, at least tangentially, to the main theme of the paper. Unfortunately, it is left pretty much to the reader to establish how this is so.

The digressions are developed at some cost to the supposed objective of the analysis. At no point does the paper provide a theory of behavior and a statement of goals, either for medical groups or for governments. In my view, no meaningful analysis is possible without these inputs. For example, it is not possible to ask whether physicians "[behave] in a self-interested way," as Professor Crichton does early in her paper, and then proceed without answering the question. It subsequently leads to much confusion concerning the discussion of professional goals, which are couched in terms like "quality control" and "protecting the consumer." Unless one has answered the original question, one cannot establish whether these are real goals, or euphemisms for financial and economic objectives.

The treatment of governments is similarly confusing. At one point, Professor Crichton seems to adopt the view that governments have been the defenders of the humanitarian ethic in Canada. I might buy this for the Saskatchewan government in 1962, but certainly not for all governments at all times. A more realistic generalization would be that governments are primarily interested in maintaining and increasing power, and do whatever is necessary and/or compatible with this goal. Among other things, this means that governments are prone to yield to pressure from the powerful medical lobby groups, unless this costs too much in terms of votes. In this context, it must always be kept in mind that professional control over medical markets has been established through government-legislated and government-enforced regulations. The profession at times may appear to be hostile to government, but ultimately must be associated with the establishment and bureaucracy that controls it. Parenthetically on this issue, there is a substantial grain of truth to the view that a professional association is an establishment-created and establishment-supported union.

Professor Crichton's view of government is the basis for her argument that a strong public bureaucracy will bring "financing and service rationing into relationship with each other." This may be a necessary condition for health policies in the general public interest, but it is by no means a sufficient condition. How to make governments more responsive to patient and consumer interests, and less sensitive to and controlled by medical association goals, is the key question, and one which, by and large, Professor Crichton has left unanswered.

NOTES

1 Elsewhere, I have discussed in some detail the dating of periods
   concerning medical policies and developments. Malcolm C. Brown,
   "The Health Care Crisis in Historical Perspective," *Canadian Journal
   of Public Health*, Vol. 70, September/October, 1979, pp. 300-306.

2 Janice P. Dickin McGinnis, "Whose Responsibility? Public Health in
   Canada, 1919-1945," p. 201-226.

MEDICAL TECHNOLOGY AND HEALTH CARE

THOMAS MCKEOWN

In a thoughtful paper published a few years ago Kass[1] drew attention to a remarkable anomaly: that medicine should be assailed by doubts about its role and purpose at a time when medical knowledge is much greater, and medical technology more powerful than ever before. Some reasons for the uncertainties are fairly obvious: the high cost of medical care and the difficulty of limiting it; questions concerning the respective responsibilities of public and private agencies for provision of health services; complex ethical issues arising from the ability to prolong, terminate, or modify life; and awkward problems of litigation which threaten to distort the face of medical practice. But there is an even more fundamental reason for re-examining the traditional approach to medical institutions, the possibility that we have misread the major influences on which health depends. Since a clarification of these influences is basic to any consideration of health strategies, I shall begin by discussing them briefly.

I

Influences on Health

An examination of the determinants of health suggests that disease arises in the following ways: (a) at fertilization, from mistakes in genetic programming; (b) in the uterus, in the course of implantation and early embryonic development; (c) after birth as a result of deficiencies (chiefly in respect of food) or hazards arising from the deficiencies (infanticide, tribal wars, etc.); (d) after birth, through exposure to environments for which the genes are not adapted. The first two may be regarded as the price to be paid for the advantages which accrue from the complex exchange of genes at fertilization and from the protection afforded by a prolonged period of intra-uterine life. The third results from man's inability to manage his environment, and the fourth particularly from failure to control his own behavior.

Against the background of these conclusions man's health history can be divided into three periods.

A. The Nomadic Period

During almost the whole of his existence man lived as a nomad, well adapted to his environment but with a short life. The main cause of sickness and early death was food deficiency, operating directly through disease and starvation, or indirectly through competition for resources which resulted in injury and death (from hunting, infanticide, tribal wars, etc.). Early man's experience of infectious disease is an open question. Living mainly in tropical and subtropical areas he no doubt suffered from vector-borne diseases, but with thinly spread populations infection was relatively less important than in the later periods.

B. The Agricultural Period

The Agricultural Revolution 10,000 years ago brought an improvement in food supplies which led to a decline of mortality and increase of numbers. The expanded populations created the conditions required by many micro-organisms and infection became the predominant cause of death. However, population growth was unrestrained, and numbers increased to the point where food supplies again became marginal. Hence the causes of sickness and death in the agricultural period resembled those in the nomadic period in that food deficiency was still critical, but differed in that micro-organisms rather than man himself presented the main threat from other living things. This change resulted from the expansion and aggregation of populations--a departure from the conditions under which man evolved--and was aggravated by defective hygiene.

C. The Transitional Period

In developed countries the past three centuries have seen a vast improvement in health and a change in the nature of the predominant health problems, from infectious to non-communicable diseases. The chief reason for the decline of infectious diseases was elimination of the conditions that had made them predominant--deficient food, uncontrolled population growth, and poor hygiene. Immunization and treatment contributed little to the reduction of infectious deaths before 1935, and over the whole period since cause of death was first registered (1838 in England and Wales), they have been less important than the other influences.

I conclude that we owe the transformation of health during the past three centuries primarily, not to what happens when we are ill, but to the fact that we do not so often become ill. And we remain well, not because of specific measures such as vaccination and immunization, but because we enjoy a higher standard of nutrition and live in a healthier environment. In at least one important respect, reproduction, we also behave more responsibly.[2] That is to say, control of infectious diseases has been achieved chiefly by modification of their origins rather than by intervention after they have occurred.

One of the most important issues concerning the future of man's health is the extent to which control of the non-communicable disease which are now predominant in developed countries will also be achieved by modification of their origins. In principle this seems possible, for few of them, and probably no "common diseases," are determined irreversibly at fertilization. But it is already evident that many of the adverse environmental influences are much less tractable than those that led to the predominance of the infections.

However when setting goals for medical research, we cannot focus attention exclusively on non-communicable diseases. In the world today there is a mix of health problems, both within countries and between countries, as diseases that were predominant in the past exist side-by-side with those that will be more significant in the future. After examining these problems I suggested that they can be divided broadly into four classes, distinguished according to the feasibility and means of their control: relatively intractable (the diseases and abnormalities determined before birth); preventable, associated with poverty; preventable, associated with affluence; and potentially preventable, not clearly related to poverty or affluence.

I concluded that in the world as a whole the predominant health problems are still those associated with poverty, and that for their solution we must rely mainly on removal of the ill effects of poverty, particularly malnutrition, defective hygiene, and excessive numbers. In developed countries, however, the chief problems are no longer attributable to food deficiency or external hazards, although these have by no means been eliminated; they are due to profound changes from the conditions of life under which man evolved. Many of these changes are in respect of behavior, facilitated by affluence--smoking, consumption of refined food, lack of exercise, etc. While clinical measures based on knowledge of disease origins will undoubtedly contribute to the

control of ill health of this type, for a solution we must rely mainly
on modification of the conditions which lead to it.

To assess the implications of these conclusions, we must consider
in turn both the non-personal services--nutrition, environment, be-
havior--on which health chiefly depends, and the clinical services--
comprising both active measures and care--which will continue to be
the central interest of the medical services. In discussing them I
will restrict attention mainly to developed countries.

II

Non-Personal Services

A. Nutrition

Although most people in developed countries have enough to eat
(their dietary health problems arise usually from excessive or ill-
balanced diets), there are, nevertheless, sections of the population
which are still inadequately, as distinct from unwisely, fed. In proportion and composition they probably vary from one country to another,
but they are mainly in two classes, the late children of large families
and elderly people, particularly those living alone.

Although there is general concern about the welfare of such
groups, they do not have the attention they would be given if it were
recognized that food is critical to their health. Nor do they receive
the kind of assistance that would be most useful, for example, food
supplements and subsidies such as were provided in many countries during
the Second World War, and whose effectiveness was reflected in health
indices in spite of deterioration in other features of working and living conditions.

Having regard for the importance of food to health, the aim of
public policy should be to use supplements and subsidies discriminating-
ly to put essential constituents within the reach of everyone, and to
provide inducements for people to prefer foods that are beneficial over
those that are harmful. Of course these aims cannot exclude all other
considerations, such as international agreements and the solvency of
farmers who have been encouraged to produce livestock and dairy products rather than grains. Nevertheless in future evaluations of agricultural and related economic policies, the health implications should
be given a primary place.

B. Environment

In their contribution to health in the past, the hygienic measures introduced progressively from the second half of the nineteenth century were second only to nutrition. However, many well-recognized risks associated with housing, atmosphere, traffic, insect vectors, and working conditions are far from being eliminated, while others inherent in contemporary life have not been fully assessed or, in some cases, recognized. In developing countries effective control of the environment has scarcely begun. In 1970 the World Health Organization reported that only 14 per cent of rural populations in the Third World had access to safe drinking water and 8 per cent had adequate arrangements for disposal of sewage.

In spite of improvements, the environment still presents many and varied threats to health. They are more complex than in the past; for example, it was easier to recognize, measure, and control the risks of infected water and polluted air than those associated with drug therapy and radiological examination of the breast. Moreover in a highly industrialized society the risks are constantly changing.

Responsibility for the environment is very fragmented, different administrations being concerned with: (a) occupation; (b) local matters, such as housing, water, and atmosphere pollution; (c) national issues such as rail, air, and road travel and pollution of seas and rivers; and (d) risks associated with medical investigation and treatment. The work associated with such large and complex problems must of course involve many administrations and professions, but it seems inevitable that there will be serious omissions so long as there is no organization, local and central, with a more comprehensive responsibility for surveillance.

I suggest that at least three steps are necessary: strengthening of the medical contribution to environmental medicine, with appropriate developments in training; a more co-ordinated approach to the different hazards in the environment--occupational, domestic, national etc.; and a considered attack on the risks associated with medical investigation and treatment.

C. Behavior

The behavioral change most significant to health in the past was
the limitation of family size which led to restriction of numbers.
This influence is critical in developing countries today, and is still
important in many developed countries which have not yet achieved a
rate of population growth consistent with the requirements of health
and welfare. Nevertheless in advanced countries it is on modification
of personal habits such as smoking, over-eating, and sedentary living
that health primarily depends.

This brings us to one of the most sensitive areas of discussion
related to health. Many people who can accept the need for public intervention in food policies, control of environment, and provision of
medical care, are deeply suspicious of attempts to modify personal behavior. Two objections are often raised: that this would be an un-
reasonable intrusion on the rights of the individual; and that any such
attempts would be certain to fail.

On the first point it is said, for example, that the individual
must be free to choose whether he wishes to smoke. But he is not free;
with a drug of addiction the option is open only at the beginning, so
that the critical decision to smoke is usually taken, not by consenting
adults, but by children below the age of consent. The question confronting society is not, therefore, whether smoking by addicts should
be prohibited; it is whether it is acceptable to induce children to become addicts at an age when they neither know nor much care about the
associated risks.

The same logic should be applied to other aspects of personal behavior which are known to be important to health. It is not suggested
that we should be required to exercise, to limit consumption of alcohol, sugar, and dairy products, and to avoid self-prescribed drugs and
some of the physician-prescribed variety, beneficial as all these measures would undoubtedly be for our health. But it is not inconsistent
with respect for personal freedom to attempt to create an environment
which encourages people to do what is good for them and to avoid what
is bad. It seems particularly reprehensible to do the reverse, to seek
ways to induce children to damage their health for no other purpose
than to sustain revenue and profits.

The conclusion that personal habits cannot be modified by acceptable public action is, I think, mistaken, and arises from the application of too short a time scale. They do change, and quite rapidly.

After all, it is not long since our ancestors were practicing infanticide, spitting on floors, tipping chamber pots into the street, and
producing large numbers of children without regard for the consequences. At the beginning of the nineteenth century no one could have
guessed that within a hundred years the most intimate of human practices, reproduction, would have been profoundly modified. And already
physicians often find themselves in company where it would be as unacceptable to light up as to spit.

However, much thought needs to be given to the means by which such
changes can be encouraged. The usual approach through advertisements,
posters, and public exhortations seems much too superficial, and takes
little account of the subtle influences which are shaping health-related behavior. There is of course no general answer to the diverse
problems associated with modification of behavior, except perhaps that
they should be considered individually and with imagination as well as
tact. Broadly what is needed is a change in way of life rather than a
commentary on it, which is all that is achieved by some of the traditional methods of health education. The examples provided by parents
to their children, by doctors to their patients, and by many of the ad-
mired figures or our time in the press or on television are some of the
most potent influences which determine behavior.

D. Evidence required for Public Action

It is sometimes suggested that action cannot be taken to modify
influences which may promote or damage health until evidence of their
effects is complete. For this reason some would say that it would be
unacceptable to change national food policies, to prohibit certain
kinds of television advertising, to control suspected hazards in industry, to restrict the use of potentially dangerous drugs, or to attempt
to modify behavior, except possibly in the case of cigarette smoking
where the grounds are considered to be sufficient.

It is fortunate that this requirement was not imposed in the past.
When Snow protected a London population from cholera in the mid-nine-
teenth century by removing the handle of the Broad Street pump, the
evidence of the relation between the disease and the water supply was
anything but complete; indeed neither micro-organisms nor tests of
significance had been discovered. If thalidomide had not been with-
drawn on the basis of an observed association between the drug and limb
deformities and when knowledge of teratogenesis was very deficient (as

it still is), many thousands of children would have been born with mal-
formations. If the argument that an association does not prove causation and only experimental evidence is conclusive had been accepted,
quite a number of people who found the relation between cigarette smoking and lung cancer sufficiently convincing would have died of the
disease before beagles had been taught to smoke. And during the last
war, if the limited foods then available had not been distributed judi-
ciously by rationing, subsidies, and supplements, the health of the
population would have been much less satisfactory than in fact it was.
Yet it was not then, nor is it now, possible to specify with any precision the nature and mode of operation of the nutritional influences
that were important.

In the light of such difficulties I believe it will often be desirable to act on the basis of high, or even moderate, probabilities,
on what has been called "a burden of prudence" rather than "a burden of
proof." When applying this principle, however, we should distinguish
between the levels of proof needed for private and for public actions.
Parents can act to protect their own or their children's health on
evidence that would not be considered sufficient to justify public action. For example, they might think it right to encourage their
children not to smoke, or to avoid white bread and to limit their consumption of foods and drinks containing sugar, at a time when none of
these practices is publicly prohibited. The level of proof needed for
public action is a different question and has no single answer. Nevertheless, it should be recognized that conclusive evidence of harm or
benefit to health is often an unrealistic requirement.

III

Clinical Services

The conclusion that medical intervention has made, and can be expected to make, a smaller contribution to health than other influences,
could not fail to have large implications for the personal health services. They have evolved on quite different assumptions; active clinical intervention is widely regarded as the basis of health and the es-
sence of medical care, and nearly half of the total health expenditure
in Britain (46.0 per cent in 1970/71) was on acute hospitals. These
hospitals do not care for most sick people, for the large majority are
in their own homes under general practitioners or in psychiatric,

geriatric, or other institutions. There are many issues which arise
from reappraisal of the determinants of health but I shall limit my
comment to some of the implications for the relationship between technology and care.

Since the eighteenth century medical activities have been divided
broadly into favored and depressed areas corresponding respectively to
patients for whom it was thought something could be done and others,
the majority, for whom little could be done. This distinction had its
origin in the admission policies of voluntary hospitals. Although
their work was not originally restricted, from the eighteenth century
it became increasingly concerned with short-term care. This made it
necessary for public authorities to accept responsibility for other
classes of patients.

In Britain the decision in 1835 to make admission to an institution a condition of public assistance brought the large number of destitute sick under the Poor Law. They were accommodated in workhouses,
supplemented later by infirmaries built as hospitals. But the infirmaries, following the example of the voluntary hospitals, restricted
their admissions, and the medical care of the indigent was left to the
mixed workhouse, the only institution unable to reject it. This group-
ing of a large heterogeneous class of patients who had in common only
their destitution was the origin of the chronic hospital.

From the nineteenth century the mentally ill, also excluded from
the voluntary hospitals, were admitted to county asylums. This separated them from the Poor Law, and led to a division of responsibility
between mental and chronic hospitals. Finally the establishment of
acute psychiatric units in general hospitals further exaggerated the
isolation of the mental hospital. The history of institutions for the
mentally subnormal is in some respects parallel. This is the background of one of the most significant features of hospitals, the separation of mental, chronic (now geriatric), and mental subnormality hospitals from general hospitals.

The distinction between hospitals had its parallel in a division
of medical practice. The founding of voluntary hospitals from the
eighteenth century, and of public hospitals from the nineteenth had two
very significant effects: it changed what had been wholly a domiciliary
service into one in which hospital work became increasingly important;
and it replaced the longstanding divisions between physician, surgeon,
and apothecary by another between general practitioner and consultant.

Originally this distinction had little justification in their training
and competence, and was determined mainly by their relationship to the
hospital. In the words of the *British Medical Journal*, a consultant
was "a practitioner among the sick who could charge higher fees because
he had a hospital appointment."

The division of medical work into favored and depressed areas
which has existed since the eighteenth century is in danger of being
extended by the growth of technology. Professional interest is increasingly absorbed by methods of investigation and treatment whose
complexities seem to challenge the attention of the best minds and
whose rewards are assumed to justify it. The acute hospital is likely
to become increasingly selective in its admission policies, and the
teaching centre with its concentration of resources and abilities will
be the most exclusive of all. Doctors, nurses, and other health workers would then be trained in an environment which reveals a very limited part of the health task, an environment where prestige, rewards, and
professional interest all seem to point in the same direction. After
qualification, understandably, they will seek to continue in the activities which were the focus of their training, and only with reluctance
will they consent to enter the massive neglected areas of health care.
The large number of patients, particularly among the congenitally
handicapped, the mentally ill, and the aged sick, whose disabilities are
not thought to provide scope for technology, will be pushed further into
the background, and the division of health services into two worlds will
be even sharper than it is today.

Many people who regret this trend, and particularly the low standards of care for the majority of patients to which it leads, nevertheless think it is justified by the achievements of acute hospitals.
They suggest that if a choice must be made, it is better to treat ap-
pendicitis in a young adult before incontinence in an elderly person.
However, such examples are quite misleading. In the first place, mean
age of admissions has risen in the past thirty years, and a comparison
between patients in acute and other hospitals is now mainly between the
old and the old, rather than between the young and the old. Secondly,
an operation which restores the patient to health is not typical of the
work of acute hospitals, much of which is palliative or unproved.
Thirdly, in what is unsatisfactorily referred to as the chronic sector,
there is scope for services which are as critical to health as those on
the acute side. Consider, for example, the need to admit to an institution a hyperactive mentally retarded child who is destroying the

health as well as the happiness of the family. Such children are to be
found in every large town; yet their care is not regarded as urgent and
is rarely given the priority it merits on health grounds.

A recent reaction to the disparity of standards is the proposal
that it should be adjusted by a transfer of resources from acute to
chronic care. However, the matter is more complex than this approach
suggests. Acute services are not all of a kind: some are among the
most effective measures that medicine can offer and any reduction of
support would be deplorable (e.g., accident services and treatment of
acute emergencies); others have never been evaluated (many surgical
procedures); still others are known to be ineffective and undoubtedly
waste resources (most tonsillectomies and, according to Cochrane,
coronary care units). What is needed is a more accurate mapping of
the effectiveness and efficiency of services, an approach more readily
applied to new developments than to existing procedures.

Moreover, the needs of so-called chronic patients will not be met
simply by an increase in expenditure, and indeed the terms acute and
chronic are themselves misleading. Patients do not fall sharply into
two classes according to their need for technology or care; those in
general hospitals need personal care; and many in mental, geriatric,
and subnormality hospitals would benefit from investigation and treatment. Furthermore, with a population of hospital patients composed
mainly of the elderly, as is the case today, the different phases of
care (acute, rehabilitative, prolonged) are often required by the same
people at different stages of their lives and sometimes at different
stages of the same episode of illness.

What is needed is a re-thinking of the whole framework of personal
services (hospitals, medical practice, and community health and social
services) in the light of the conclusion that the task confronting the
services is the complete care of patients, using that term in the wid-
est sense to include active rehabilitation, prolonged and terminal
care, as well as investigation and treatment of acute illness. In
broad terms what is required is a framework which meets, and where
necessary reconciles, the diverse needs of technology and care. This
aim is unlikely to be achieved under a fragmented hospital system which
isolates the majority of patients (mental, geriatric, and subnormal)
from the resources of the general hospital, or in a system of medical
practice in which the hospital work of the general practitioner is
separated (in community hospitals) from the work of the consultant.[3]

IV

Prevention, Technology and Care

Perhaps the most basic problem confronting health services is to strike a judicious balance between three activities: the prevention of disease by personal and non-personal measures; investigation and treatment of disease; and the care of the sick who need personal attention but no longer provide scope for active measures. I think there is little doubt that until now medical interest and resources have been focused on the second area and, to a lesser extent, on personal prevention by immunization. The other responsibilities for non-personal preventive measures and for long-term care and terminal illness have been relatively neglected.

When considering the distribution of effort between these activities, planners should feel for the present and think for the future. We cannot trust the motives of some who can ignore present suffering when preparing a blueprint for the future; but we also cannot trust the judgment of others who are overwhelmed by existing problems and give no thought to what is to follow. So, while it is wholly to the credit of a parent that he will think that any expense is justified in treatment of his sick child, an administrator who acts solely on the assumption, without regard for the effectiveness or efficiency of the service, will make very poor use of the available health resources.

The improvement in health during the past three centuries was due essentially to provision of food, protection from hazards, and limitation of numbers, and assessment of the residual health problems suggests that the same influences are likely to be effective in the future. But with this difference, that in developed countries personal behavior (in relation to alcohol, diet, exercise, tobacco, drugs, etc.) is now even more important than provision of food and control of hazards. It follows that if health is to improve substantially, increased attention must be given--in education, research, and services--to the non-personal measures which are the predominant determinants.

In clinical services the provision of acute care will continue to be predominant, for it is a response to what the patient usually considers to be his most urgent need. But this service does not justify the place it has occupied hitherto in medical thought and practice. It is sometimes extremely effective, and when it is it justifies the fullest support; but it is often ineffective, or tides the patient over a short illness leaving the underlying disease condition and prognosis unchanged. There is therefore need for adjustment, in priorities and relationships, between technology--using that term to cover a wide range of active measures--and care.

NOTES

1 L. R. Kass, "Regarding the end of medicine and the pursuit of health," *The Public Interest*, 40 (Summer, 1975), p. 11.

2 T. McKeown, *The Role of Medicine: Dream, Mirage or Nemesis?* Second edition, Princeton University Press, 1979.

3 I have described the kind of hospital that would need these requirements in *Medicine and Modern Society* (London: George Allen and Unwin, 1965).

COMMENT ON THE PAPER OF MCKEOWN

CATHY CHARLES

In numerous articles and books, Dr. McKeown has developed an important conceptual framework of the major determinants of health and
policy directions for improving health. In his paper, "Medical Technology and Health Care," presented at this conference, Dr. McKeown
summarizes this conceptual framework. There are several themes which
are central to his overall argument and I would like to begin by identifying three of primary importance.

1. Historically, the major factors contributing to a decline in mortality from infectious diseases in England and Wales were improved nutrition, better hygiene, and the introduction of contraceptive measures,
i.e., changes in the conditions which gave rise to disease. Medical
interventions such as immunization and treatment contributed little to
the reduction of infectious diseases prior to 1935 and, even after,
were less significant than these other non-medical influences.

2. In industrialized societies, non-infectious diseases have now replaced infectious diseases as the major health concerns. Significant
breakthroughs in controlling these problems will also depend on effecting changes in the conditions which give rise to them--environmental
factors and personal behaviors.

3. The major thrust of the health care system, with its emphasis on
acute care hospitals, high technology intervention, and fragmentation
of types of care, is misdirected. What is needed is a framework of
personal services which emphasizes the complete care of patients, a
closer alignment of various components of the health care system, and
a reconciliation of the diverse needs of technology and care.

Because Dr. McKeown's arguments are critical of medicine, it is
sometimes assumed that his perspective is similar to that of Ivan
Illich[1] and other medical critics of this genre. This is not the case,
and it is instructive to point out some of their differences. Dr.
McKeown's approach is predominantly that of the historical epidemiolo-
gist. He has undertaken a detailed empirical analysis of the relative
impact of medical interventions on the decline in mortality from infectious diseases and his criticism of medicine's contribution in this

regard derive from this analysis. It is not the medical profession as
an institution which Dr. McKeown challenges, but rather the predominant
mechanistic model of disease-supporting therapeutic intervention.
Illich, on the other hand, criticizes the medical profession as an institution of immense power, influence, and social control. The medical
profession, according to Illich, does more harm than good for both patients and society, a conclusion which Dr. McKeown would be unlikely to
reach.

Several reviewers of Dr. McKeown's writings, while accepting his
basic conclusion (as I do) that major improvements in health status in
the past derived predominantly from modifications of the origins of
disease, rather than from intervention after they occurred, nonetheless
challenge the means by which this conclusion is reached and some of its
implications. There is some validity to these concerns.

First, Dr. McKeown's assessment of the relative unimportance of
medical intervention in controlling infectious diseases is based primarily on the argument that such interventions contributed little to an
overall decline in death rates from infectious diseases. There is a
danger here in relying too much on mortality statistics. These do not
reveal the impact of medical intervention on changes in patterns of
morbidity and hence may underestimate the importance of therapeutic intervention. In addition, there are numerous methodological problems
associated with the interpretation of trends in mortality statistics
over a time-frame stretching from the mid-1800s to the present.

Second, even if medical interventions have not been as important
as other influences, it does not follow that these have been unimportant or are now unimportant. A reading of the first edition of Dr.
McKeown's *The Role of Medicine*: *Dream, Mirage or Nemesis*,[2] on which
much of this paper is based, easily leaves the impression that the
author is critical of the clinical function. Dr. McKeown attempts to
correct this impression in his preface to the second edition.[3]

Finally, some critics, while agreeing with Dr. McKeown's interpretation of the past, nonetheless disagree that future improvements in
health status will derive primarily from modifications in the conditions giving rise to disease, rather than to modifications in disease
processes. The logic of Dr. McKeown's argument is similar whether applied to the past or future. What has changed is the nature of currently predominant diseases and the major conditions fostering them.
Chronic diseases have replaced infectious diseases as the primary

health problems in developed countries, and these are fostered by more complex environmental conditions and unhealthful personal behaviors.

I would agree with Dr. McKeown that over the long run, changing these conditions offers great potential for improving health status but, in the short run, organized attempts to modify unhealthful personal behaviors are likely to be hampered by a lack of both proven techniques for effecting change and successful program models. This means that many diseases which may now in theory be preventable are not so in practice. The burden on the health care system to intervene in such cases will remain acute. Even where prevention does succeed, one major effect may be to shift rather than relieve pressures on the health care system, for improvements in the quality and duration of life effected through preventive measures will likely postpone rather than eliminate the need for various types of health and personal care services.

The view that more emphasis should be placed on modifying unhealthful behaviors associated with disease and less emphasis placed on disease intervention has gained increasing popularity in recent years. The Canadian Lalonde report, *A New Perspective on the Health of Canadians*,[4] which reflects Dr. McKeown's work, was a major influence in promoting this view. What this means for the medical profession is presumably an expanded or at least redirected role, such that physicians are expected to assume a broader responsibility for health care and to act to some extent as "change agents" attempting to alter individual lifestyles and behaviors in healthy ways. There are strong forces both within and outside the medical profession urging physicians to take on this broader role. This is reflected in the introduction of a variety of "behavioral science" courses in medical school curricula and in exhortations to physicians to treat the whole patient, taking into account social and psychological factors rather than simply focusing on disease.

There is, however, an alternative view expressed by such writers as Conrad,[5] Zola,[6] Kittrie,[7] Pfohl,[8] Divoky and Schrag,[9] Freidson,[10] and others, who see inherent dangers in the expansion of medical influence over personal behaviors. These writers argue that the power of the medical profession to redefine or relabel as illness an increasingly wide range of attitudes and behaviors has grown at an alarming rate and cite examples such as drug addiction, alcoholism, learning disabilities, a variety of compulsive behaviors, and child abuse. This trend

is seen as problematic for reasons which relate directly to the theme
of this conference. The "medicalization" of an increasing number and
range of behaviors is viewed as greatly expanding the medical profession's influence to encompass not only a broader role in diagnosis and
treatment, but also the right to redefine our very notions of health
and illness and to impose increasingly narrow limits on the range of
acceptable behavior. Moreover, it is argued, the labelling process
itself may foster negative consequences for the individual through a
process of stigmatization.

I raise this issue not to argue for or against the views expressed,
but rather to highlight the strong and divergent opinions currently
held regarding an expanded role for physicians. On the one hand, there
is a strong push for physicians to devote more attention to encouraging
individuals to alter unhealthy behaviors associated with disease, or
which themselves are thought to be diseases. On the other hand, there
are those equally adamant who oppose expansion in the profession's influence over such behaviors. My own view is that physicians and other
health professionals should play an important role in encouraging individuals to reduce "risk factors" which have been clearly associated
with specific diseases. What is harder to define is the total range of
behaviors and problems over which medical influence should be encouraged and the appropriate limits and forms which such intervention
should take.

A final issue which I wish to highlight relates to what Dr.
McKeown has described as the major failures in the orientation of
health care services in Britain today. He argues that attention is
focused on acute care and high-technology intervention with relatively
low priority given to the alignment of different components of care and
to major groups in society requiring long-term care. He makes the important point that the institutional separation of high-technology and
personal care fails to meet the needs of patients who may require both
types of services. The rapid growth in technology reinforces these
trends and contributes to an imbalance in services between favored and
depressed areas.

These problems are not unique to Britain. Similar concerns have
been expressed about the organization of health care in both Canada and
the United States. It is interesting to note that these three health
care systems have different origins in terms of political philosophy,
the role of government, and the financing of health care services. But

despite cross-national variations in these dimensions commonly thought
to influence the operation and thrust of health care systems, the major problems identified in the provision of services across countries
are remarkably similar. A possible explanation for this trend is that
the application of professional norms and knowledge and the increasing
role of health care technology transcend national boundaries and are
leading to a convergence in problems faced by different health care
systems.[11] Whether this will also lead to a convergence in the types of
solutions adopted is an interesting question for the future.

In this commentary I have been able to discuss only a few of the
many provocative and insightful issues which Dr. McKeown raised in his
paper. I have tried to focus on those of particular importance to the
theme of this conference. Dr. McKeown has been a dominant figure in
re-orienting our conceptual thinking about the major determinants of
health, and in so doing he has made an extremely important contribution.

NOTES

1 Ivan Illich, *Medical Nemesis* (Toronto: Bantam Books, 1977).

2 Thomas McKeown, *The Role of Medicine*: *Dream, Mirage or Nemesis?*
   First edition (London: The Nuffield Provincial Hospitals Trust,
   1976).

3 Thomas McKeown, *The Role of Medicine*: *Dream, Mirage or Nemesis?*
   Second edition (Princeton: Princeton University Press, 1979), p.
   vii.

4 Marc Lalonde, *A New Perspective on the Health of Canadians* (Ottawa:
   Information Canada, 1975).

5 Peter Conrad, "The Discovery of Hyperkinesis: Notes on the Medicalization of Deviant Behavior," *Social Problems* 23 (1975), 12-21.

6 Irving Kenneth Zola, "In the Name of Health and Illness: On Some
   Socio-Political Consequences of Medical Influence," *Social Science
   and Medicine* 9 (1975), 83-87; "Medicine as an Institution of Social
   Control," *The Sociological Review*, New Series 20 (1972), 487-504;
   "Healthism and Disabling Medicalization," in *Disabling Professions*,
   Ivan Illich et al., eds. (Great Britain: Marion Boyars, 1977).

7 Nicholas Kittrie, *The Right to Be Different* (Baltimore: Johns
   Hopkins Press, 1971).

8 Stephen J. Pfohl, "The Discovery of Child Abuse," *Social Problems*
   24 (1977), 310-321.

9 Peter Schrag and Diane Divoky, *The Myth of the Hyperactive Child*
   (New York: Dell Publishing Company, 1975).

10 Eliot Freidson, *The Profession of Medicine* (New York: Harper and
    Row, 1970), pp. 244-278.

11 For further discussion of this theme, see John Colombotos, Catherine
    Charles, and Corinne Kirchner, "Physicians' Attitudes Toward Politi-
    cal and Health Care Policy Issues in Cross-National Perspective: A
    Comparison of FMG's and USMG's," *Social Science and Medicine*, 11
    (1977), 603-609; E. C. Hughes, *The Sociological Eye*, Vol. 2 (New
    York: Atherton, 1971), p. 386; David Mechanic, "The Comparative
    Study of Health Care Delivery Systems," in *The Growth of Bureaucrat-
    ic Medicine*: *An Inquiry into the Dynamics of Patient Behavior and
    Organized Medical Care*, Ch. 2 (New York: John Wiley, 1976), pp. 23-
    48.

CONCLUSION

DONALD E. LARSEN

Some readers of this volume may experience the same type of ambivalence that was expressed at the concluding session of this Workshop when some individuals in effect said: "While some papers were informative, provocative, and novel, it was difficult to grasp the meaning or intent of other papers and to identify linkages between some papers, especially in terms of the conference theme."

Such impressions are to be expected at a conference which brought together both academicians and practitioners from a variety of disciplines and employment settings to consider the problem of power and authority in medical care. Under these circumstances it is inevitable that the papers would present the reader with different theoretical perspectives, modes of expression and vocabularies, levels of abstraction, time perspectives, types of intellectual craftsmanship, and attitudes and values vis-à-vis the Workshop theme.

Although exposure to such diversity may be bothersome to some, it has the potential benefit of stimulating individuals to consider the problem at hand from new perspectives and to strive for clearer communication with persons from other disciplines. Of course, it can be annoying to observe that seminal works in one's own discipline go unnoticed by members of other disciplines. However, multi-disciplinary conferences can help to direct attention to new sources of thought and thereby possibly diminish the intellectual isolation that characterizes many disciplines.

What themes, or common issues and problems, were raised in the papers presented in this volume? What conclusions can be drawn from them? An individual's answer to these questions is apt to be influenced by the well-known psychological mechanism of "selective perception," that is, the tendency to view the world selectively as a result of personal experiences, interests, and conditioning. This principle was aptly demonstrated by four of the Workshop speakers[1] who, by prior arrangement, had agreed to offer their observations of the conference proceedings at the concluding session. The selectivity of their perceptions is suggested by the fact that there was little duplication in

what each speaker viewed as the major issues or themes in the papers.
Such individual differences undoubtedly exist as well among readers of
this volume.

My own selective interpretation is that a major concern of the
papers was the description and analysis of the relationship between
social change and the shifting patterns of power and authority in medical care. More specifically, it seems to this writer that the papers
either implicitly or explicitly addressed four questions: (1) What
changes have occurred in the relative distribution of power and authority in medical care? (2) What forces in society have influenced these
changes? (3) Of what social consequence are the changes? (4) How can
the existing balance of power and authority be deliberately changed?

Before commenting on the authors' answers to these questions,
there are three points that should be made about their approaches to
the questions. First, most of the authors did not define the terms
"power" and "authority" or distinguish between these concepts. Indeed,
some did not use these terms explicitly, but only implicitly. Nevertheless, the two terms were typically used to refer to what Elliott
Krause, a sociologist, has simply described as "...the ability of one
individual or group to compel another group to do something which the
compeller wants done, whether the compelled wants to or not."[2] Only a
few authors followed the common practice of restricting the use of the
term "authority" to power that is legitimized by virtue of office or
law.

Secondly, two of the papers (by Roy and McKeown) focused on power
and authority of the *institution* of medical care, while the reference
point of the other authors was power and authority of specific *roles*
and *role players* (e.g., doctors, nurses, patients). The power and
authority of the doctor was a major preoccupation of the papers. Only
the nurse, among more than 100 types of health-related occupations in
existence today, received more than passing attention.

Finally, all but two of the papers concentrated on twentieth-century medical care; the remaining two (by Mitchell and Gelfand) dealt
with the origins of modern-day medicine in eighteenth- and nineteenth-
century France. Despite the different historical context of the latter
papers, they nonetheless dealt with questions about the nature, sources,
and consequences of *change* in physicians' power and authority. From an
abstract point of view, the social processes to which they refer are
similar to those described in the other papers. However, it was not

their intention to comment on the dynamics of change in the twentieth
century and therefore the two papers are not referred to in the following comments.

1. Patterns of Change

Change in the character and direction of power and authority in
medical care is one of the major themes in the collection of papers in
this volume. The complex, dynamic, and divergent nature of this change
presents a challenge to the reader who wishes to discern patterns of
change in twentieth-century medicine. This task is further complicated
by the fact that some authors simultaneously describe changes that have
occurred, make evaluative judgments about the changes, and prescribe
other changes that should take place.

Patterns of change in medical power and authority presented in
this volume can usefully be discerned in terms of the three bases of
physicians' Aesculapian authority which were cited in Moskop's paper:
sapiential authority ("medical expertise"), *moral* authority ("acting in
the best interest of patients"), and *charismatic* authority ("interpersonal influence").

Two contrary trends in medical sapiential authority are referred
to in this volume. As described most vividly in Roy's paper, modern
medicine is amassing through biotechnological advances enormous power
on matters relating to prolonging or terminating life and in the emerging area of genetic engineering. Similarly, other papers refer to the
widening influence of medicine over behavioral problems as a result of
the expanded definition of appropriate medical concerns.

These examples of growing medical influence are contrasted with ,
the present-day realization, enunciated clearly in McKeown's paper, of
modern medicine's relative powerlessness in coping with the major ills
of our day, such as cancer, heart disease, accidents, and mental illness. On balance, then, a very mixed picture of trends in sapiential
authority is presented in this volume: enhanced powers in some areas
of medical expertise, but diminished abilities to influence the course
of prominent contemporary health problems.

It is in the areas of moral and charismatic authority that medicine's traditional position of influence has eroded in recent decades,
according to various accounts in this volume. The transformation of
health institutions into a position of "domination" over their clientele, as posited by Weidman, is one illustration of the declining moral

authority of medical institutions and their personnel. The relative decline of physicians' traditional moral authority at the patient-care
level is exemplified in the papers by Herbert, Flaherty, and Freedman.
The papers by McGinnis and Crichton refer to the diminished power of
physicians to act on behalf of patients' interests in government policy-
making circles. Finally, numerous references in the papers to publicly
expressed criticisms and doubts about medicine and medical care are
symptomatic of a declining charismatic medical authority. Such expressions signify a reduction in the traditionally high levels of respect
and esteem accorded to physicians, which in turn undermines charismatic
authority.

Taken as a whole, the papers in this volume describe a relative
decline in traditional medical authority, notwithstanding the signs of
increased medical power in some domains of treatment. Reactions to
diminishing medical authority are mixed. The two papers by physicians
(Hatfield and McLeod) leave little doubt that the medical community is
alarmed by the trend, for reasons which will be considered later. Only
the paper by Moskop explicitly offers qualified approval of the changing pattern of medical authority. This paper, however, is careful not
to endorse the radical position of Illich or Szasz, who advocate a
greatly diminished role in society for physicians and medical care.

2. Sources of Change

The authors are particularly detailed in their efforts to account
for the decline in medical authority in North America, and by extension, in industrialized western countries in general. They join a long
list of other analysts who have been on a similar quest.[3] A close look
at their accounts reveals a complex web of socio-political-technologi-
cal factors--too complex to elucidate and unravel easily here. However, it should be stressed that the authors' search for the sources of
change draw our attention to forces within the institution of medical
care (e.g., rising medical technology, bureaucratization of medical
care, professionalization and proliferation of health occupations, mis-
placed emphasis on curative medicine, patient alienation, medical education, etc.) and to broader societal changes (e.g., demographic shifts,
including rising levels of education, growth of egalitarianism, growing
influence of government, the questioning of basic institutions, rising
expectations, etc.). A persistent theme underlying these analyses is
the suggestion that physicians in particular and medical care

institutions in general have either not recognized or are not adequately responsive to changes that are buffeting them both from within and
outside their traditional domains of influence. For their part, however, physicians at this Workshop expressed concern that medicine is
being unjustly criticized and blamed for this state of affairs in medical care and stated that physicians alone should not be held accountable.

3. Consequences of Change

Few of the papers in this volume actually address themselves to
the question of the impact, either positive or negative, of declining
medical authority in society. Some papers refer to the declining mor-
ale and relative incomes of physicians, which are very real by-products
of diminishing authority. Other papers (Moskop and McLeod) express
concern about the deleterious impact on medical care that may arise
from an erosion of physician authority. On the other hand, some authors (Moskop, Flaherty, and Freedman) see benefits for both patients
and other members of the health team stemming from a re-allocation of
power to these parties. Indeed, the health benefits that are thought
to arise from increasing the responsibilities and powers of patients
are a motivating force behind the patients' rights movement, referred
to in several papers.

4. Bringing about Change

A number of papers refer to methods that may be effective in ma-
nipulating the balance of medical authority. Some authors were moved
to consider this question because of their desire to shift power either
to patients or to members of the health care team other than physicians.
Whatever their goal, the authors typically propose "solutions" that
follow logically from their diagnosis of the causes of the decline in
authority. Thus, Weidman advocates the replacement of a unicultural
perspective in health care with a more responsive transcultural perspective as one method of bolstering the effectiveness of medical care
institutions. A greater emphasis on accountability is seen by Flaherty
and McLeod as a necessary and effective way to boost the authority of
nurses and physicians. McKeown proposes that greater authority for the
institution of medical care will only come about through a major shift
in the emphasis of its activities, namely, from curative to preventive

care. This shift will occur, he says, only with a realignment of our
thinking about disease causation.

As these examples suggest, efforts to change the balance of power
and authority in medical care will require major shifts in the thinking
and behavior of doctors, patients, and society. The authors have provided a glimpse into the complexity and challenge of this task.

NOTES

1 Drs. Flaherty, Mitchell, Moskop, and Weidman.

2 Elliott A. Krause, *Power & Illness: The Political Sociology of
   Health and Medical Care* (New York, 1977), p. 225.

3 See, for example, Bernard R. Blishen, *Doctors & Doctrines*, *The
   Ideology of Medical Care in Canada* (Toronto, 1969); Eliot Freidson,
   Professional Dominance: The Social Structure of Medical Care
   (New York, 1970); John H. Knowles, ed., *Doing Better and Feeling
   Worse: Health in the United States* (New York, 1977); and David
   Mechanic, *The Growth of Bureaucratic Medicine* (New York, 1976).

Also published by Wilfrid Laurier University Press
for The Calgary Institute for the Humanities

RELIGION AND ETHNICITY
Edited by Harold Coward and Leslie Kawamura

Essays by: Harold Barclay, Harold Coward, Frank Epp, David Goa, Yvonne Yazbeck Haddad, Gordon Hirabayashi, Roger Hutchinson, Leslie Kawamura, Grant Maxwell, Cyril Williams

1978 / pp. x + 181 / ISBN 0-88920-064-5 / **$5.00** (paper)

THE NEW LAND
Studies in a Literary Theme
Edited by Richard Chadbourne and Hallvard Dahlie

Essays by: Richard Chadbourne, Hallvard Dahlie, Naïm Kattan, Roger Motut, Peter Stevens, Ronald Sutherland, Richard Switzer, Clara Thomas, Jack Warwick, Rudy Wiebe

1978 / pp. viii + 160 / ISBN 0-88920-065-3 / **$5.00** (paper)

THEORIES OF PROPERTY
Aristotle to the Present
Edited by Anthony Parel and Thomas Flanagan

Essays by: C. B. Macpherson, William Mathie, David Daube, Susan Treggiari, Anthony Parel, James Tully, John Pocock, James Moore, James MacAdam, Nannerl Keohane, Douglas Long, John Gray, E. K. Hunt, Tom Settle, Thomas Flanagan, Shadia Drury

1979 / pp. viii + 395 / ISBN 0-88920-081-5 / **$8.00** (paper)

SCIENCE, PSEUDO-SCIENCE AND SOCIETY
Edited by Marsha P. Hanen, Margaret J. Osler, and Robert G. Weyant

Essays by: Paul Thagard, Adolf Grünbaum, Antony Flew, Robert G. Weyant, Marsha P. Hanen, Richard S. Westfall, Trevor H. Levere, A. B. McKillop, James R. Jacob, Roger Cooter, Margaret J. Osler, Marx W. Wartofsky

1980 / pp. x + 303 / ISBN 0-88920-100-5 / **$7.50** (paper)

CRIME AND CRIMINAL JUSTICE IN EUROPE AND CANADA
Edited by Louis A. Knafla

Essays by: J. H. Baker, Alfred Soman, Douglas Hay, T. C. Curtis and F. M. Hale, J. M. Beattie, Terry Chapman, André Lachance, Simon N. Verdun-Jones, T. Thorner and N. Watson, W. G. Morrow, Herman Diederiks, W. A. Calder, Pieter Spierenburg, Byron Henderson

1981 / pp. v + 339
ISBN 0-88920-098-X / **$9.50** (paper)
ISBN 0-88920-118-8 / **$15.00** (cloth)